ISBN 9781734768701
ISBN 9781734768725
Printed in the United States of America

Book design by Je'Mahl D. Ray
Edited by Jennifer M. Ray

Table of Contents

Introduction

Dedication

Endorsements

(African, Mediterranean, Asian, Western)

INTRODUCTION

We're living in a ever changing world. Overwhelmed by technology ,career and family commitments, our wellbeing has taken the backseat. Generally, we are all very familiar with the concepts and purposes of "food" and "eating. However, do we really understand bio-sustenance or food biology?

Most people will answer "no". In the era of fast food and quick fixes, we've become disconnected from what truly nourishes us.
If you're like me, and have always pondered these questions, you're in the right place.

My name is Malaika Bagoudou. I am an Integrative Nutrition Health Coach, personal chef, and an author. As a holistic health coach, I mentor busy families with a hands-on approach to inspire a balance within with work, home and other social demands. Together, we create a healthier, simpler, and more enjoyable life. As every client's needs are unique, I fashion your individual health history, personality, and goals into a easy plan that fits your lifestyle.

A little bit about my personal story:

There came a time in my life where I was completely exhausted by the vast collection of health advice out there. From fad diets and fitness gurus telling me what to eat and how to take care of the body to contrasting opinions, I became discouraged. Then I asked myself, "Why am I listening to what everyone else is doing and not feeding my body based on what I need?
As the old wise saying goes: "One man's food could be another one's poison"! So, I made a decision that changed my entire life: I became an Integrative Nutrition Health coach. I learned which lifestyle and nutrition changes I needed to make to bring my body back into balance.

I healed myself from a thyroid disease and removed unnecessary weight, permanently. The programs I implement with my clients are not necessarily diet-focused. The entire person is the focus - mind, body and spirit. This method determines which of your body's systems endure the most strain. My mission is to help busy men and women and their families triumph over their health issues, maintain a healthy lifestyle, or even wipe the slate clean.

In addition to my work as an IN Health Coach, I also specialize in hair and skin care. This collective alone has truly helped me understand the link between what we put in our bodies and internal /healthy health.
My formal education includes:
 - The Institute for Integrative Nutrition
 - Formula Botanic School
    - Texas Central College of cosmetology

My priority is to help every client unleash the healing power within! Are you ready to dive in?
For more information on my programs and services please view my website @ www.Lesgrainesdevie.com and start exploring.
I can't wait to see you taking the lead on your fantastic health journey. For now, let's get cooking, shall we?

Dedication

I dedicate this cookbook to all the busy families across the globe especially military members and their families; thank you for your service.

To all of my family especially my husband Yao Bagoudou, my son Daniel and my daughter Abigail Bagoudou for your thorough love, patience and unlimited support, I love you; you have made this journey an easy one .

To my Mentors, Je'Mahl and Jennifer Ray and their children. Thank you for all your timeless support and dedication from the early stages of my dream.

To all my Moms and dads who God blessed me with across the globe, you inspired me to soar high and I am grateful. My friends who have been there since the beginning until now, thank you for your support and encouragement.

My parents, especially my mother who initiated my passion for cooking since an early age, you have undoubtedly inspired me to enjoy creating with flavors and color. To my uncle who allowed me to use his kitchen as my lab, l am very appreciative for your generosity.

To my heavenly Father the one and only, who shaped me from my mother's womb and bestowed upon me many gifts and talents, to you be the glory for ever and ever.

Endorsements

I'm a Certified Integrative Nutrition Health Coach... who.... really enjoys cooking!! I admit it!!! Between coaching, and other roles as an author and speaker, and developing online programs and affiliate programs, and trying to incorporate other important aspects of life, well, I literally am too busy to cook! Or so I thought!

Malaika's soul shines through this wonderful cookbook. The visuals are amazing. The recipes are quite easy! The first one that caught my eye was Togolese Peanut Butter Soup with Collard Greens! Then, African Mushroom Coco Curry. Oh! And the Artichoke Panache and Cauliflower & Corn Rice. So many tantalizing recipes!

Here's the thing: Any time I see a three-step cooking process, I'm IN! I can handle it!!!

Malaika – thank you so much for creating this wonderful gem of a collection! It's a tremendous help to people like me who are Too Busy To Cook!!!

- Lynn DelGaudio,
Integrative Health Coach, Author, Speaker, www.lynndelgaudio.com

Chef Malaika helped me identify the right foods to eat for my thyroid disorder and then meal plan. Quick healthy whole-food meals that my entire family will eat!

_Amber Hood, military wife and mom of 4.

Healthy food has never taste so good! There is not one dish I've had from Les Graines de Vie that I do not love!

-Leti

Chef Malaika's meals are the ultimate balance between simplicity and excitement. Meals that remind you of home but with unmatched flavor! She's served many events with friends and family and people cannot stop complimenting her recipes!

-Margaret Sullivan

Les Graines de Vie 's food is so good it makes me want to dance! Every dish is full of flavor.

-Jerome

Your "Lab"
The Kitchen

Having a nice environment to explore your cooking ideas is vital. A organized kitchen is part of a healthy relationship with food. We ea with our eyes first. Food and cooking are both memories. Let's mak every dish memorable. Now, let's get organizing, shall we?

6

Pantry Makeover 101

Organizing your pantry is necessary in order to easily see all the resources you have at your disposal. It will also save you money during grocery shopping and time during cooking prep. Organization is the key to successful healthy living and eating.

Now, are you ready to enjoy cooking?

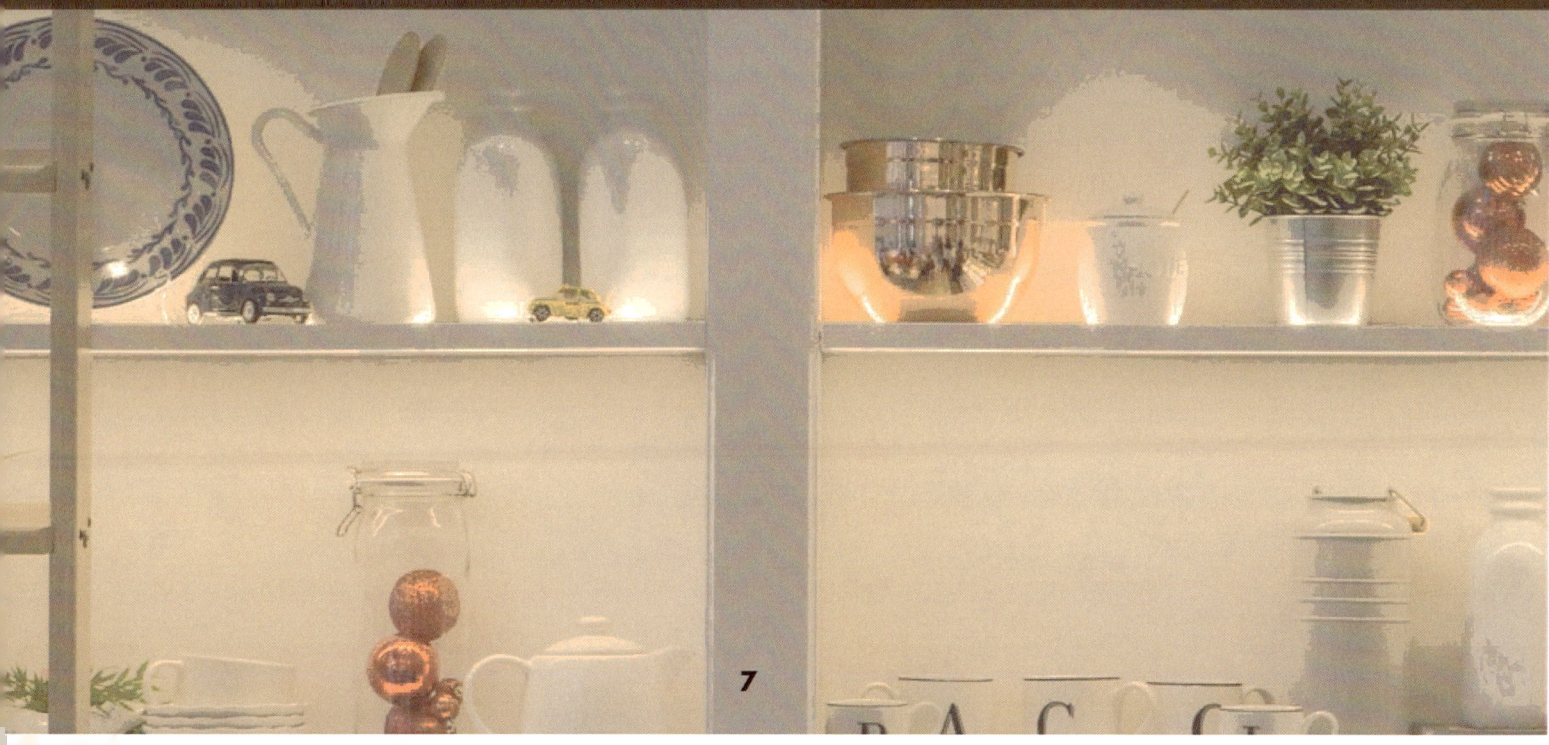

Cooking Bases, Marinades, and Sauces

What are they?

Cooking bases are mixtures of ingredients like herbs, spices, or broths in a concentrated blend in order to enrich the flavor of the food.
Marinades are mixtures of oil, spices, and acids such as lemon juice, which helps break down the enzymes for a great flavor on the inside as well as the outside. vinegar, wine used to enhance the flavor of food. The acids help tenderize meats

Sauces are seasoned liquids or semiliquid mixtures that are used as condiments or added to the food while cooking. They provide flavor, add color, and help moisturize the food.

Why do you need them in your kitchen?

I'm glad you asked, they provide great flavor as well as vital nutrients. In order to enjoy your food, the flavor must be present.
I make them ahead of time and store them in my refrigerator. Posing as efficient way to make quick and easy meals in no time. Saturdays are great days in my household to do my meal planning for the week. Doing this saves a lot of time, and encourages you to make healthy meals for your family throughout the week. It makes life a breeze! For now let get cooking , shall we?

JERK CHICKEN BASE

Ingredients

4 bunches fresh thyme
  leaves
½ cup chopped scallion
½ tsp black pepper
1 green jalapeño
2 cloves garlic
½ cup water

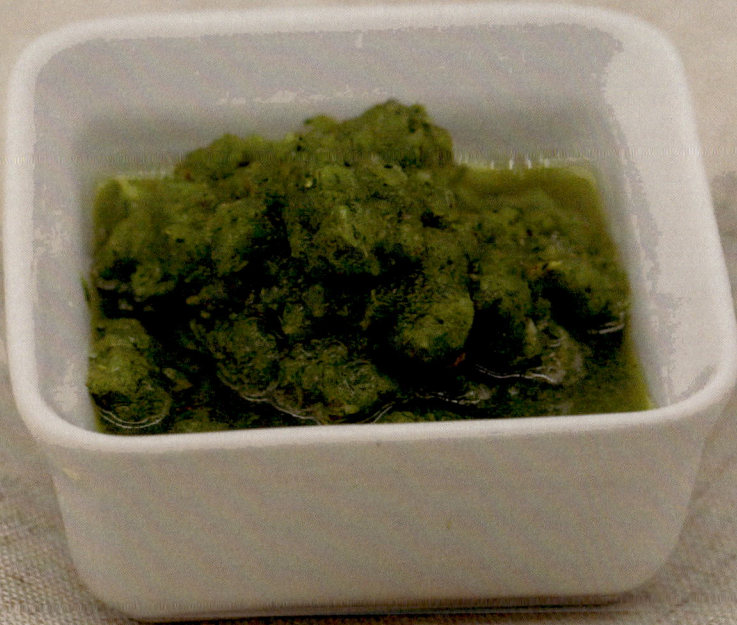

Directions

1 In a blender or food processor, add thyme, scallion, black peppers, jalapeño, garlic, and water.

2 Blend all the ingredients to a smooth consistency.

3 Store the mixer into a clean air tight container in the fridge and use it as a base (marinade) for jerk chicken

This base can stay in the fridge up to two weeks.

Herbs and spices have a powerful benefit for your health. They are not just packed with flavor but are also boosting agents for your immune system.

TOGOLESE HOT SAUCE "YEBESE"

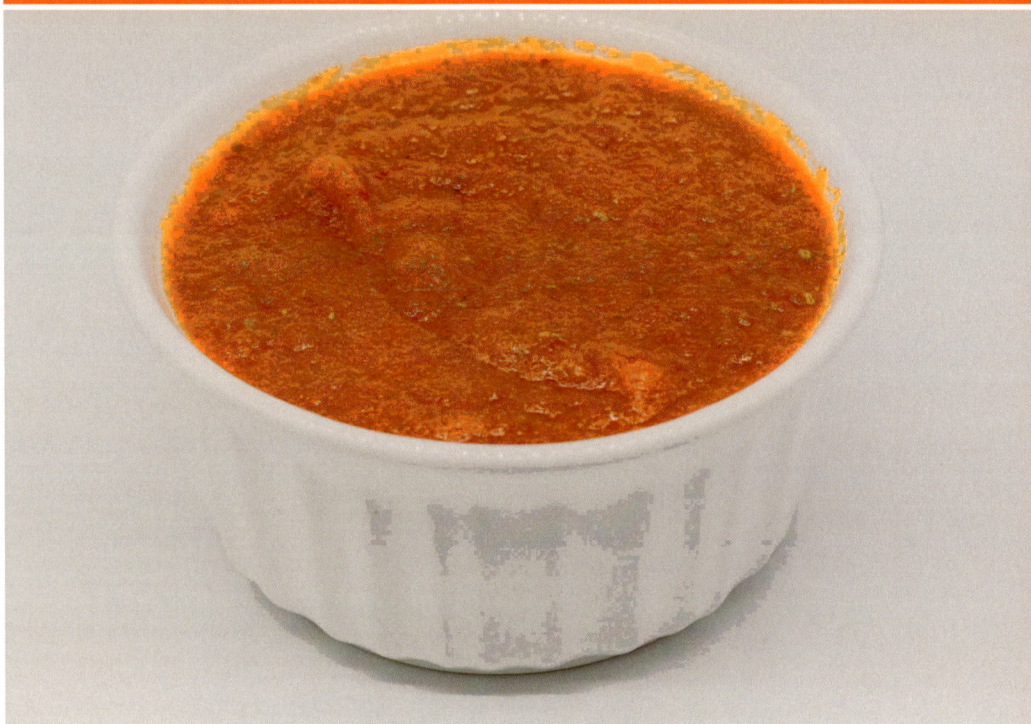

5 minutes and multiple uses

Ingredients

5 habanero peppers
I medium onion cut
3 cloves garlic
1 medium tomato
1 tbsp bouillon powder or stock
¼ cup olive oil
1 tsp kosher salt
1 tbsp smoked paprika
1 tbsp dried oregano
½ cup water

Directions

1 In a food processor, add habanero peppers, onion, garlic, tomato, bouillon powder, salt, smocked paprika, oregano and water.

2 Blend all the ingredient to a smooth paste.

3 In a medium heat sauce pan, add oil and the blended mixture.
Let the mixture cook for 3 minutes, then reduce the heat and simmer it for 5 more minutes until the water is absorbed. It will be a thick paste when all water get's absorbed.

This sauce pairs well with Togolese black-eyed pea fritters, Yummy! It can also b used as a base for any stew that requires hot pepper. Refrigerate the sauce up to three weeks.

Adding hot pepper to your diet i a heart-healthy choice. It may also help with weight loss (belly fat burning agent).

Mirepoix Base

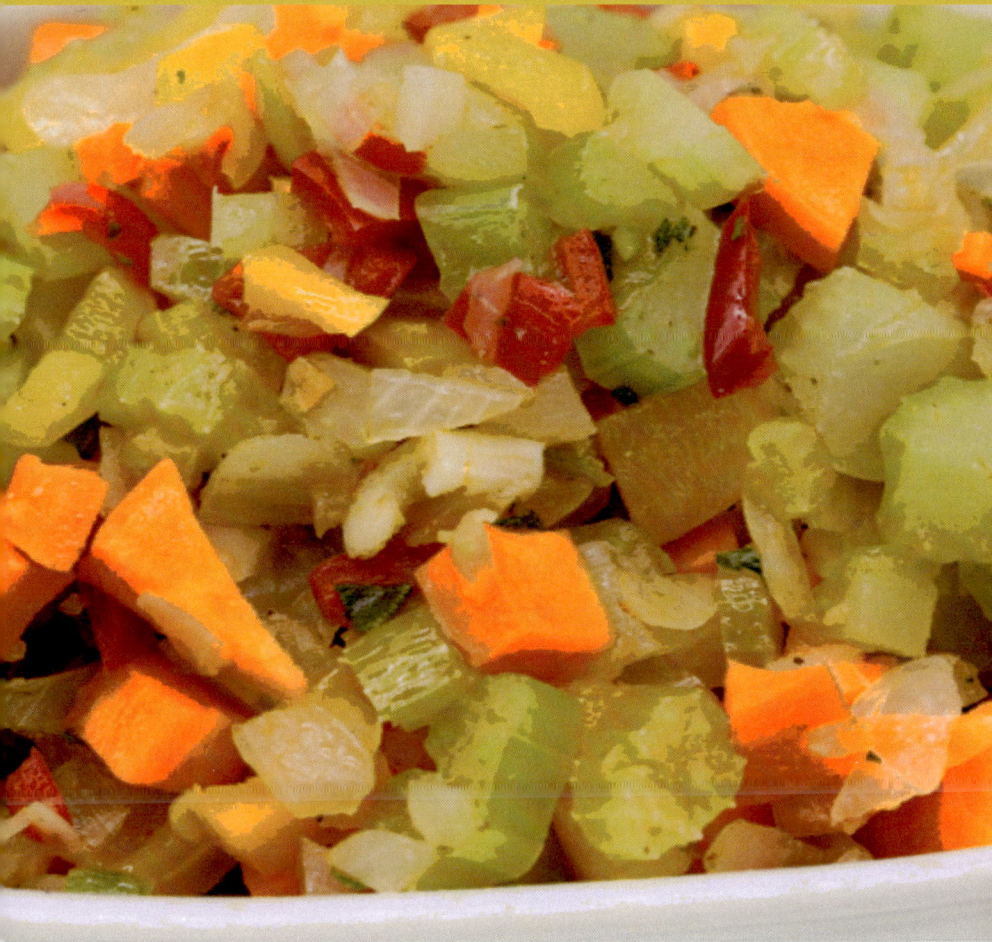

Ingredients

4 cups diced white onion
2 cups diced celery
2 cups diced carrot
2 tbsp Irish butter or olive oil
3 cloves garlic ½ cup diced
    red bell peppers (optional)
½ yellow diced bell peppers
    (optional)

Mirepoix is a flavor base made from vegetables that are cut into small pieces and then cooked with butter, fat, or oil in a low heat over a long time.
Having French as my First language, I was introduced to a mixture of Togolese and French cuisine at an early age. Mirepoix is one of my favorite ones. Mirepoix can be used for stocks, sauces, soups or stew.

Directions

1 In a medium sauce pan, heat butter   to mcdium and add garlic, celery, carrot, onion, to the pan. Lower the heat and cook the veggies for 8 minutes or until translucent or soft.

Rich in flavors but also packed with vital nutrients, vitamins and minerals like beta-carotene, antioxidants and vitamin C

Classic Rub Sauce

Ingredients

2 tbsp olive oil
1 tbsp Düsseldorf mustard (German
1 tsp coarse ground Dijon mustard
1 tbsp smoked paprika
1 tbsp chipotle spice
1 tbsp rice vinegar
1 tbsp dried minced onion
2 cloves garlic grated
1 tsp miso paste or tamarin sauce
1tsp kosher salt
1 tsp black pepper
1 tsp dried oregano

Mustard has the ability to speed up the metabolism, and stimulate digestion.

Directions

1 In a medium bowl, add the mustards, paprika, chipotle spice, rice vinegar, minced onion, garlic, meso paste, salt, black pepper, dried oregano and olive oil.

2 Take a wire whisk and stir the mixture very fast for about 3 minutes until all elements are well incorporated.

3 Store the rub sauce into a clean glass jar and refrigerate for future use.

Bell Pepper Garlic Base

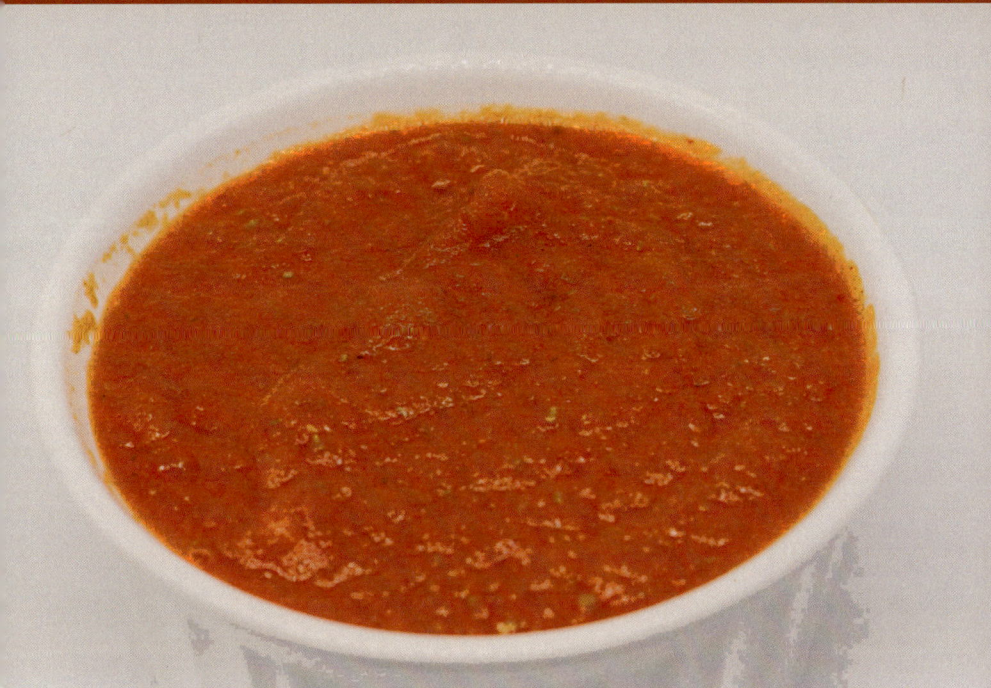

This base can be used as marinade by adding salt or stock. Or, just a simple base to make stews.
To tenderize meat, add 1 tbsp vinegar, and 2 tbsp olive oil.

Ingredients

1 medium red bell pepper
1 medium yellow bell pepper
1 chili pepper
6 cloves of garlic
1 medium onion (red)
1 tbsp tarragon
1 tsp smoked paprika
1 tbsp rosemary

Bell peppers are packed with a variety of vitamins and antioxidants. They have the ability to improve eye health.

Directions

1 In a blender or food processor, add bell peppers, chili, garlic, onion, tarragon, smoked paprika and rosemary.

2 Blend the ingredients until they congeal into a thick and smooth paste.

3 Store the mixture into an air tight glass jar. Use it as marinade, stew base or soup base.

Anise Seeds, Ginger, Thyme

This base is suitable for fish and poultry.
You can also use it as a base for stews, soups, and casseroles.

Directions

1 In a food processor, combine ginger, anise seeds, onion, peppercorn, garlic, thyme and water.

2 Blend the ingredients to a smooth and pasty texture.

3 Pour the mixture into a glass jar and store it in the fridge for up to 3 weeks

Ingredients

¼ cup fresh grated ginger
2 tbsp anise seeds
1 medium onion
1 tsp peppercorn
3 cloves garlics
2 fresh thyme leaves
½ water

Spices are power houses for nutrients. Spices like anise, and ginger help with digestion, and may reduce inflammation.

Pesto Sauce

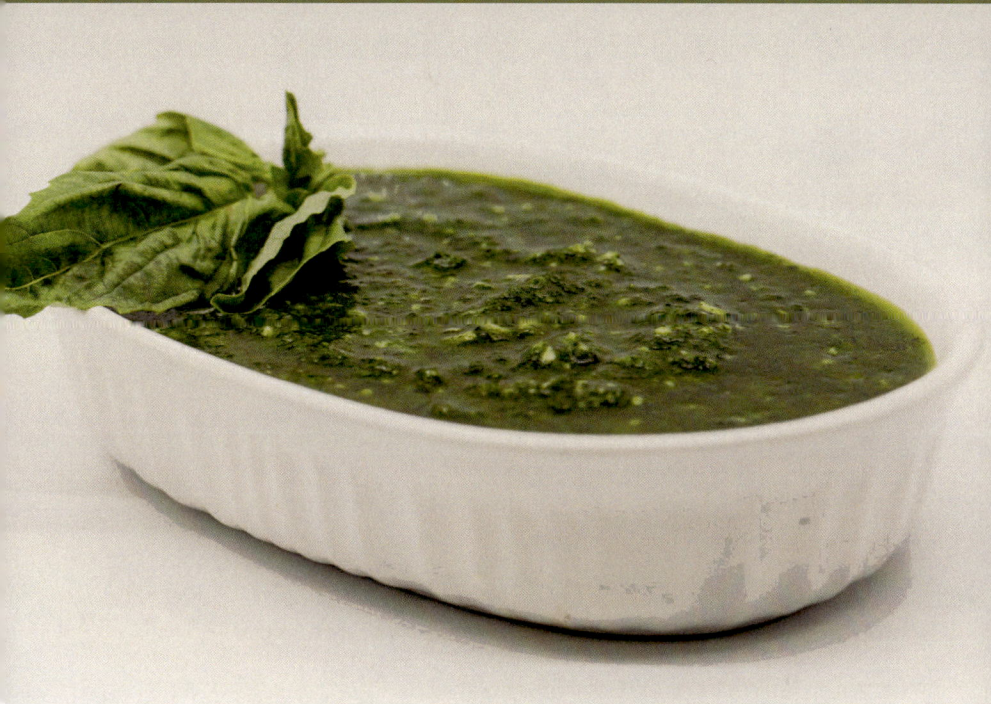

10 minutes and multiples uses

Ingredients

2 cups shopped curly parsley
1 cup fresh spinach shopped
1 cup olive oil
4 cloves garlic
1 tsp kosher salt
1tsp stock powder (LGDVB)
   or any stock
1 ¼ cup Parmigiano-Reggiano
   cheese
½ cup water

Directions

1 In a food processor or blender, add parsley, garlic glove, spinach, olive oil, salt and pulse a couple of times, add cheese, stock powder (LGDVB), water and blend the mixer to a creamy consistency.

2 Pour the sauce over fettuccine or store it in an air tight glass jar in the fridge for future use. It lasts about 4 -5 days.

This fresh pesto sauce is the real deal, from consistency to flavor.
Pesto is also great for meat, fish, poultry and vegetables. Delicious!

Parsley is the main ingredient in this pesto, rich in nutrients and vitamins such as A, C and K. It is a great antioxidant agent.

*LGDVB (Les Graines De Vie Bouillon

15

Home made Bouillon

Salsa de Fresca (Pico de Gallo)

Ingredients

1 cup diced roman tomatoes
1 diced jalapeño pepper
1 cup diced red onion
½ cup diced yellow bell peppe
1 tbsp lemon juice
1 tsp kosher or Indian salt
2 bunches fresh parsley choppe

Directions

1 In a medium bowl, add the tomatoes, jalapeño, red onion, yellow bell pepper, lemon juice, 1 bunch parsley chopped and salt.

2 Mix all ingredients together. Taste the salsa to ensure the degree of hotness and flavor,

3 Serve the salsa with your favorite chips or crackers.

This salsa is fresh. It can also be used in making omelets. If you are allergic to tomato, use diced zucchini and mix bell peppers instead. Yummy! It is easy to make and fresh.

Tomatoes are rich in Vitamin C, potassium, folate and Vitamin K. They are a great source of antioxidants.

Dressings & Vinaigrettes

What are they?

Well let's find out, Vinaigrettes are mixtures of oils and acids element like lemon juice, vinegar or wine. They are use to dress salads or
marinate meat , fish or vegetables for a strong flavor with combination with spices and fresh herbs.
Dressings on other hands are simples sauces that usually cold but are used to top salads, fresh vegetables, meat dishes and fish for a perfect flavor. Dressings can have as base oil, vinegar, mustard, avocado, sesame seed butter, mayonnaise, and yogurt. The list go on.
I personally like to try with anything that has a creamy consistency.
A vinaigrette is a type of dressing, but not all dressings can be called vinaigrettes. The benefit of making your own is that you can control what goes on your dressings or vinaigrette. Anytime you make one from home, you just save yourself from a lot of foods additives, salts and chemicals. Once you start making your own, I guarantee you won't go back to stored-bought! For now let get cooking shall we?

Honey Lemon Dijon Vinaigrette

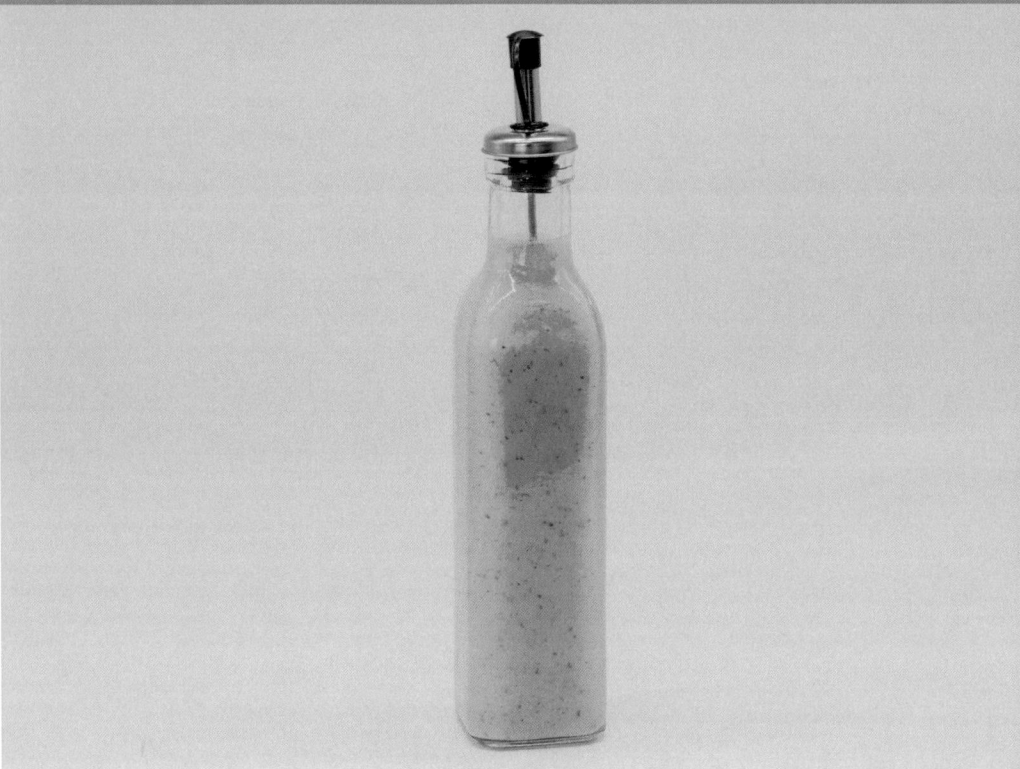

Ingredients

1/2 cup extra virgin olive oil
3 tbsp rice vinegar or apple
   cider
   vinegar
½ tsp black peppers
1 tbsp lemon juice.
1 tsp pure honey
1 tbsp Dijon mustard
1 tbsp Düsseldorf mustard
   (German)
   Pinch of salt

*This mouthwatering
vinaigrette will shift the way
you add salad into your diet.
It's fresh and simple
You have to give it a try.
It can also be used to
marinate meats.*

Directions

1 In a blender or food processor, add all the
ingredients and blend to a creamy consistency.

2 Store the vinaigrette in an air tight glass bottle
and refrigerate for future use. It can last up to
two weeks.

*Making your own vinaigrette
is a simple and active way to
ensure you have control of
what goes into your system.
Store bought vinaigrettes
have a lot of additives that
are harmful to health.*

Chipotle Vinaigrette

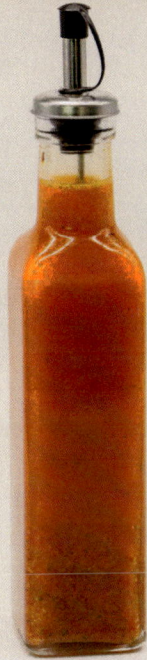

Ingredients

1 tbsp chipotle spice (seasoning
2 tbsp olive oil
1 tbsp rice vinegar
½ tsp kosher salt
1 tsp Dijon mustard
1 tsp tamarin sauce
1 tsp garlic powder
1 tsp onion minced
1 tsp miso paste
1 hot cherry pepper

Directions

1   In a blender or food processor, add all the ingredients and blend well to a running consistency.

2   Store the vinaigrette in an air tight glass bottle and refrigerate for future use. It can last up to two weeks.

This vinaigrette is wholesome, simple, yet delicious.
Made with real ingredients and
suitable for marinating meats, poultry, or seafoods.

Making your own vinaigrette is a simple and active way to unsure you have control of what goes into your system. Store bought vinaigrettes have a lot of additives that are harmful to health.

Sesame Seed Ginger Vinaigrette

Ingredients

2 tbsp tahini
1 tbsp tamarin sauce
1 tbsp grated ginger
1 clove grated garlic
½ cup sesame oil
1 tbsp lemon juice
1 tbsp Dijon mustard
4 tbsp rice vinegar
½ tsp spicy brown mustard

Directions

1 In a blender or food processor, add all the ingredients and blend to a creamy consistency.

2 Store the vinaigrette in an Air tight glass bottle and refrigerate for future use.

*Note: It can last up to two weeks.

Making your own vinaigrette is a simple and active way to ensure you have control of what goes into your system. Store bought vinaigrettes have a lot of additives that are harmful to health.

*This delectable vinaigrette is a must on your DIY bucket list.
It's as easy as A-B-C!*

5 Minute Breakfast bowls

Healthy Eating

Breakfast just like it sounds, "break the fast", it's the first meal of the day. Breakfast jumpstarts your metabolism.
I am not an early breakfast eater but, I do consistently enjoy good breakfasts .
Why is it so important to have a healthy breakfast?
Healthy breakfast in the morning is the least you can give yourself before starting your day.
Tremendous studies have proved that children who don't eat breakfast in the morning may have insufficient minerals, fiber, and important vitamins. These vital nutrients help children perform better in school.
I do believe that most of the time, the reasons why people skip breakfast is a lack of time, lack of easy access to healthy food, and a lack of motivation. Sometimes the lack of motivation is actually an old habit that carried over from childhood.
From my own experience, being born and raised in Togo, West Africa, where cooking food is enlaced in our culture, I can say that my parents had engraved the skills into me since early age. I'm very glad that they did.
Eating a healthy breakfast:
Boosts your energy by refilling your glucose in the morning.
Provides essential nutrients, minerals and vitamins in order to keep your body functioning property.
May reduce the risk of diseases.
Most of the time when we skip breakfast, we tend to eat a large meal at lunch, trying to compensate.
That's why this book is just what a busy person or parents needs. It packed with quicks delicious recipes. For now let get cooking, shall we?

Fruity Oatmeal Bowl

Ingredients

1 cup old fashion oats
2 tbsp dry powdered milk or
    coconut powder
1 tbsp raw honey
1 cup mixed fruit (red
    raspberry, blueberry,
    blackberry, or strawberry)
1 tbsp coconut flakes
½ cup milk (regular or plant
    based milk)
1 cup hot water
1 tbsp hemp seeds

To make this breakfast bowl vegan, use coconut powder and coconut milk instead. The color of this dish is so compelling…
"We eat with our eyes first."

Oats are one of the healthiest grains on the planet. Rich in fiber, minerals, vitamins, and antioxidants.

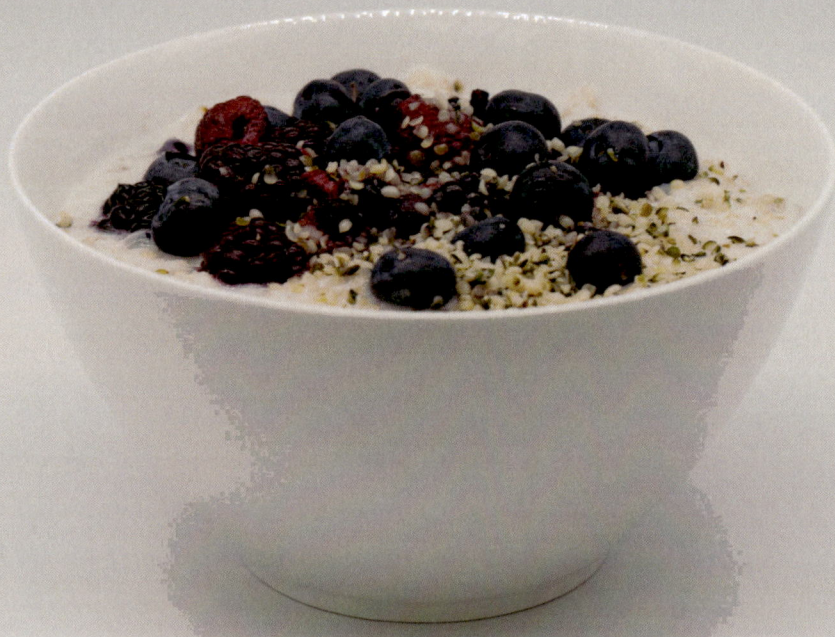

Directions

1 In a bowl, add oats and water, mix well with a spoon and microwave for 3 minutes.

2 Remove from the microwave, combine milk powder and milk or coconut milk, honey and mix well until all elements are well incorporated to a smooth consistency.

3 Top it with fresh mixed fruits, coconut flakes, hempseed and enjoy!

Wholesome Brown Rice Pudding

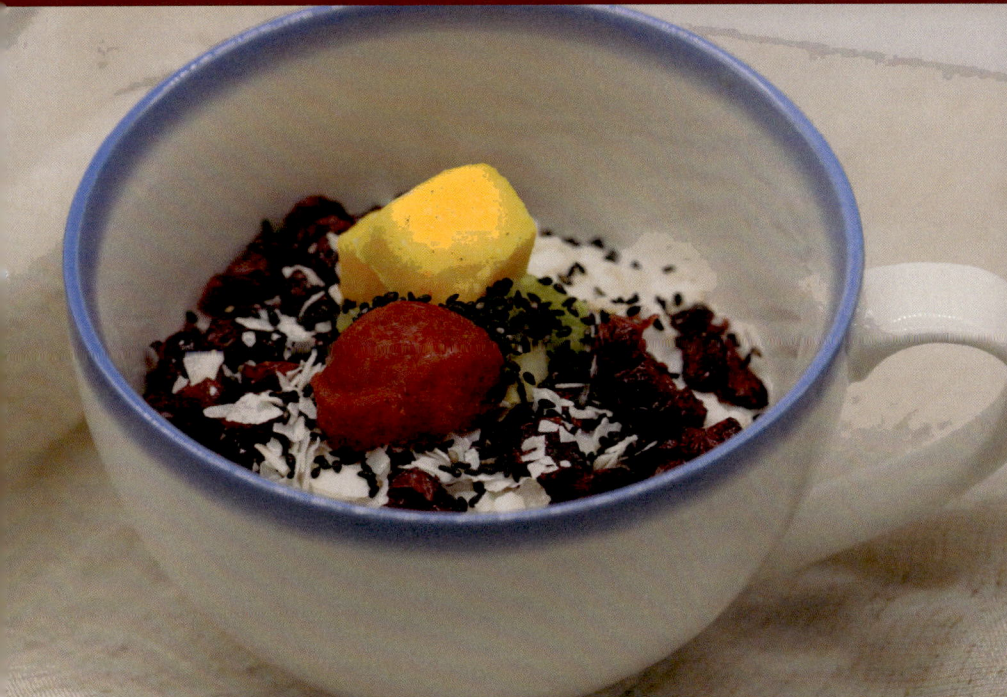

Ingredients

1 cup cooked brown rice
1 tsp caraway seed
3 tbsp vanilla Greek yogurt
1 tbsp organic coconut flakes
1 tbsp dried cranberries or
    combination of raisin and
    nuts
2 cubed mango
1 strawberry
2 slices of kiwi

Directions

1   In a cup or a cereal bowl combine brown rice and yogurt. Give a good mix until all is well coated.

2   Add kiwi, dried cranberries, coconut flakes, caraway seeds. Top with mango and strawberry. Enjoy!

3   It can also be refrigerated for one hour as a nice cold desert.

A breakfast in under 10 minutes is a must for those rushing in the mornings. This one is a wholesome food for the body!

This pudding is very satisfying because of the fiber content in brown rice. It's a healthy dessert or breakfast without added Sugar.

Degue' Couscous "aka' Couscous Pudding

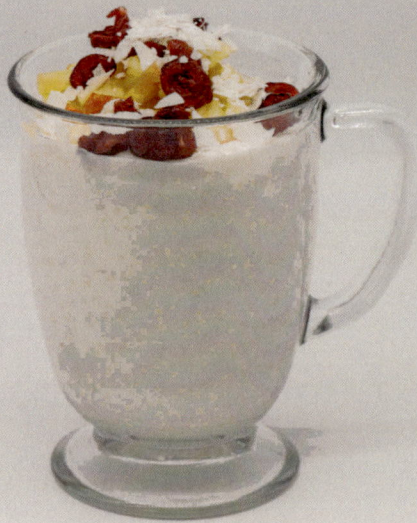

Ingredients

1 cup cooked couscous
3 tbsp vanilla Greek yogurt
¼ medium apple cubed
2 tbsp cranberry
1 tbsp coconut flakes

Directions

1   In a cup, combine couscous, yogurt, and give a good mix until all is well coated.

2   Top it with coconut flakes, and dried cranberries, fresh cubed apple, or raisins.

Enjoy! It can also be refrigerated for one hour as a nice cold desert.

Couscous is a low calorie grain made of Durham wheat Semolina. Couscous is rich in fiber, protein, vitamins and minerals.

Couscous is a staple food in North Africa.
This pudding is very delicious and filling. For vegan diets, use coconut yogurt instead.

Blissful Morning Avocado Smoothie Bowl

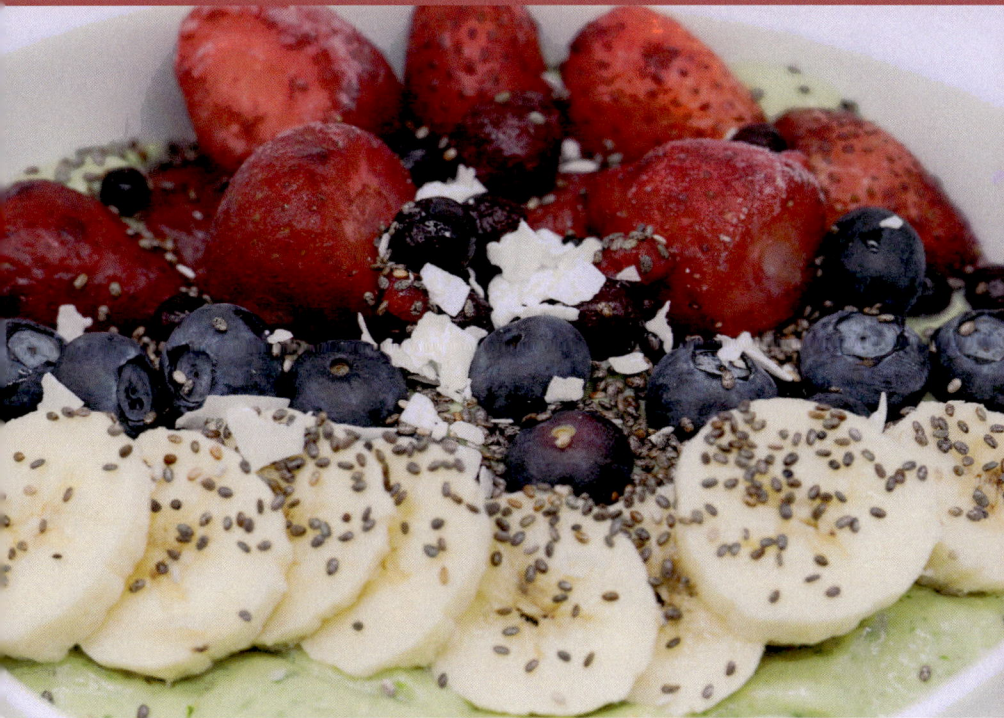

Ingredients

2 small ripped avocados cut and peeled

2 tbsp vanilla Greek yogurt or coconut cream

1 tbsp chia seeds

1 cups mix berries (strawberries, blueberries, and black berries)

1 tbsp dried coconut flakes

1 cup whole milk or coconut milk

1 big banana cut in half

1 tsp pure honey

1 tsp flaxseed meal (ground)

1 cup fresh or frozen kale/ spinach

Directions

1   In a food processor or blender, add peeled avocado, half banana, and Greek yogurt, whole milk, honey, flaxseed meal and kale.

2   Blend all the ingredients to a creamy and smooth consistency.

3   Serve the smoothie in a bowl.
Top it with mixed berries, cut the half left of the banana in thin round slices,
Add the banana slices to the bowl and sprinkle   coconut flakes on top. Enjoy!

A luscious smoothie ready to boost your energy in the morning!
This double potassium smoothie is a must for your morning routine.

Avocados are high in healthy fats, and rich in folate. Eating avocado in moderation may help to maintain a healthy weight.
Did you know that avocados are fruits?
Amazing Right! There was an old saying in Africa, that avocados look like the belly of a pregnant woman, therefore good for expecting mothers.
Do you know some facts about avocados?

Unforgettable Pro-Fiber Bowl

Ingredients

2 tbsp creamy peanut butter
3 tbsp cottage cheese
1 medium banana sliced
¼ cup strawberries,
¼ apples slices
¼ mango cubed
1 tsp pure honey
1 tbsp coconut flakes
  (optional)
1 tbsp dried cranberry
1 tbsp chia seeds

Directions

1 In a clean bowl, add peanut butter, cottage cheese, banana slices, strawberries, apple slices, kiwi, and mango cubed.

2 Sprinkle dried cranberry, coconut flakes on top with chia seeds, and drizzle honey over the mixture.

3 Before you take your first bite, stir everything thoroughly for a nice consistency and enjoy!

Almond butter is another great substitute for this bowl. To make it vegan, use coconut yogurt instead of cottage cheese.

This bowl is a complete protein & fiber. Suitable for boosting energy!

Glorious Green Toss

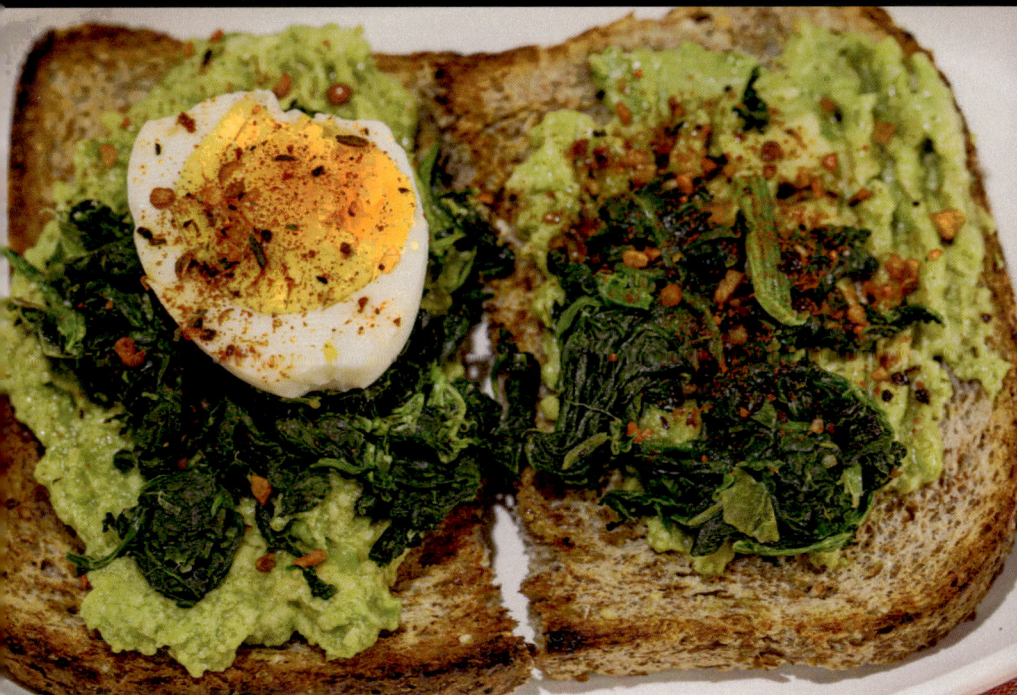

Ingredients

2 toasted slices of Ezekiel
    Sprouted Grain Bread
1 ripened avocado
1 boiled egg
1/2 cup of baby spinach
1 tbsp of ghee butter
Dash of red pepper flakes
¼ tsp kosher salt
1 tsp garlic powder

For the creamiest consistency, the avocado can be drizzled with a little olive oil for a healthy ration of Omega 3 and 6.

Ezekiel bread is high in protein and contains a lot of amino acids, topped with avocado. It is a great source of Vitamin A, C, E, K, and B-6.

Directions

1 In a small bowl, peel the avocado, add salt and mash it to butter consistency.

2 Turn the stove to a medium heat, in a pan, add ghee butter, and let it melt for 2 seconds, then add baby spinach. Cook the spinach for about 2 minutes. Add salt, and garlic powder.

3 In a tray, spread the avocado butter over the bread, add the spinach and top it with the boiled egg, then dash the red pepper flakes and enjoy!

Savory Oatmeal rice bowl

5 minutes 1 serving

Ingredients

1 cup whole grain quick oat
1 ½ hot water
1 tsp Indian black salt
1 tsp garlic powder
1tsp red pepper flake
2 tsp chipotle seasoning
1 tsp smoked paprika
1 large sunny side up fried egg
1 tbsp avocado oil or olive o

Directions

1 In a medium glass or cereal bowl, add oat and pour the hot water. Give it a quick stir and microwave for 2 minutes.

2 Remove from the microwave , add oil, salt, garlic powder, chipotle seasoning, smoked paprika and stir very well until all the ingredient are incorporated.

3 Top the savory oatmeal rice bowl with the sunny side up fried egg and a sprinkle of black pepper and enjoy!

This dish is a replacement for those morning rice bowl Delicious but yet packed wit. a lot of fiber. Instead of regular oatmeal with Sugar. eat this and taste the savory unique flavor it brings.

Oats are one of the healthiest grains on the planet. Rich in fiber, minerals, vitamins and antioxidants

Under 15 Minute Dinners:

Healthy Salads

Salads are light and have a reputation of being a low calorie food and are high in fiber.

Incorporating salads into your diet is a better way to control weight.

Salads can be served as a side dish or a meal by paring them with proteins.

Spring Mix & **Pomegranate**

Ingredients

3 cups spring mix salad
1 medium cucumber rounds
    slices
½ cups cherry tomato halves
6 pieces dates shopped
1 tbsp hempseed (culinary
    grade)
3 tbsp sesame seed ginger
    vinaigrette
2 tbsp Ariel of pomegranate

Pomegranate is considered a superfood. They contain anti oxidants and vitamins. Great fruit for healthy eating!

Digestion starts with our eyes, this exquisite salad will mesmerize your eye sight and make your taste buds jump a first bite.
You have to taste it and see!

Directions

1   In a large bowl, add spring mix, cucumber, cherry tomatoes.
    Top the salad with shopped dates, and pomegranates.

2   In a large bowl, add spring mix, cucumber, cherry tomatoes.
    Top the salad with shopped dates, and pomegranates.

3   Toss the salad couple times to ensure that the vinaigrette is evenly distributed.

Classic Mediterranean Salad

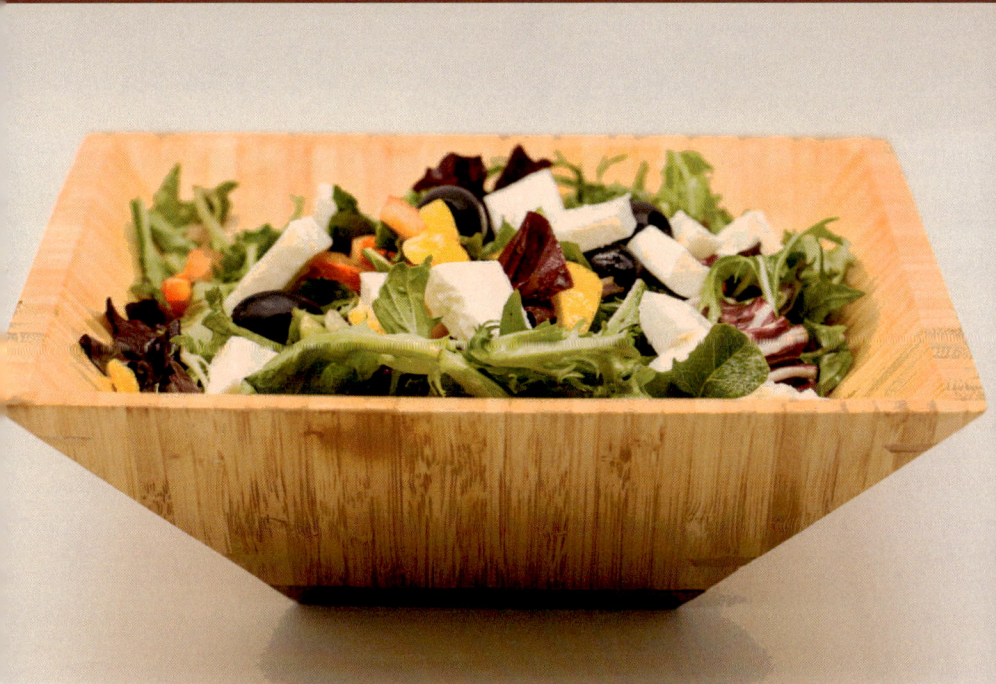

Ingredients

3 cups fresh spring mix (24 OZ)
½ cup black olive
1 Roma tomato julienne cut
1 medium yellow bell pepper (julienne cut)
½ cup cubed fresh mozzarella
3 tbsp honey lemon Dijon vinaigrette

Directions

1 In a large bowl, add spring mix, Roma tomatoes, bell pepper, and black olives.

2 Top the salad with fresh Mozzarella and drizzle vinaigrette.
Toss the salad a couple times to ensure that the vinaigrette is evenly distributed.

3 Serve the salad with one protein or grain of your choice & enjoy!

This classic Mediterranean salad is colorful and simple, yet delectable. To make this salad vegan, omit the mozzarella cheese.

Quinoa Panache'Bowl

15 minutes and 4 servings

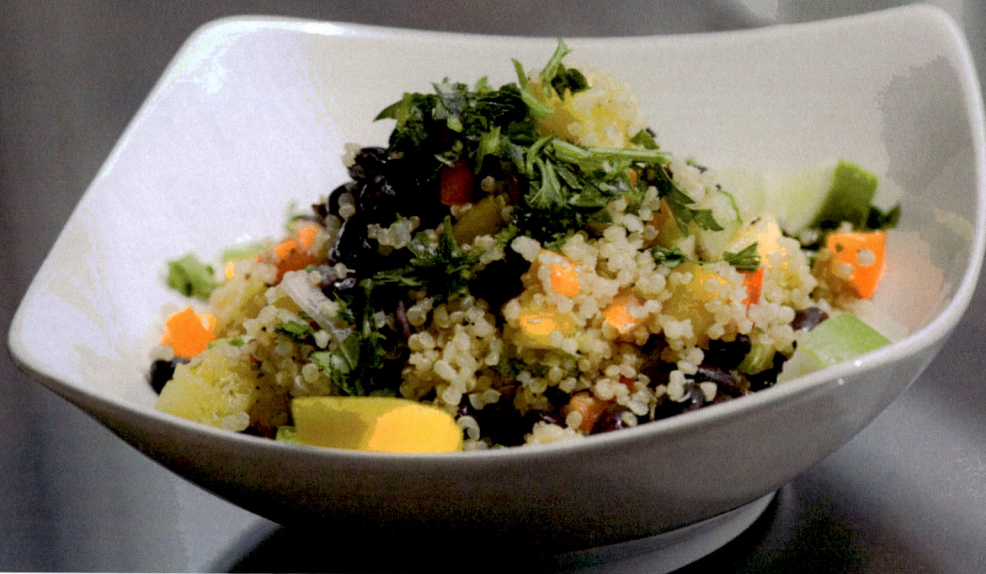

Ingredients

I can black beans
2 cups Quinoa
½ zucchini cubed
1 cup mixed bell pepper
    cubed (yellow, orange, and
    red)
2 bunches fresh parsley
2 tbsp Chipotle vinaigrette or
    Rub sauce
½ cup plum tomato halves
¼ medium red onion cubed

Directions

1   Place the quinoa in a fine-mesh strainer and rinse under cold water for 2 minutes.

2   In a medium saucepan, combine the rinsed quinoa, water and salt. Bring to a boil. Reduce the heat to low and cover the saucepan with a lid. Simmer for approximately 15 minutes.

3   Remove the pan from heat and let it rest for 5 minutes. Remove the lid and fluff the quinoa.

4   In a big bowl, combine quinoa, cubed mixed bell peppers, red onion, black peppers, zucchini cubed, plum tomatoes, black beans and chipotle vinaigrette. Mix well and serve.

Top it with fresh parsley and enjoy!

*To make this dish even faster, have the quinoa pre-cooked or make ahead.
It's also a great option for vegetarian and vegan diets. It can be accompanied with baked fish or chicken.*

Quinoa is a whole grain, rich in protein. It's loaded in fiber rich also in iron, and magnesium.

Butternut Squash Salad

Ingredients

1 cup butternut squash seeded
    peeled and cubed
    Spring mix salad
10 cubed Feta cheeses
1 cup mixed red & yellow bell
    peppers (julienne cut)
1 tbsp olive oil
5 sticks Chow Mein noodles
    (optional)
3 tbsp chipotle vinaigrette

One can't have enough greens on their palate, paired with a scrumptious vinaigrette, it's Heaven on Earth!
Did you know that: Chow Mein noodles are a crunchy complement to any meal or salad in traditional Asian Cuisine?
Now you know, try it!

Leafy greens like spring mix are power houses for fiber, minerals and vitamins.

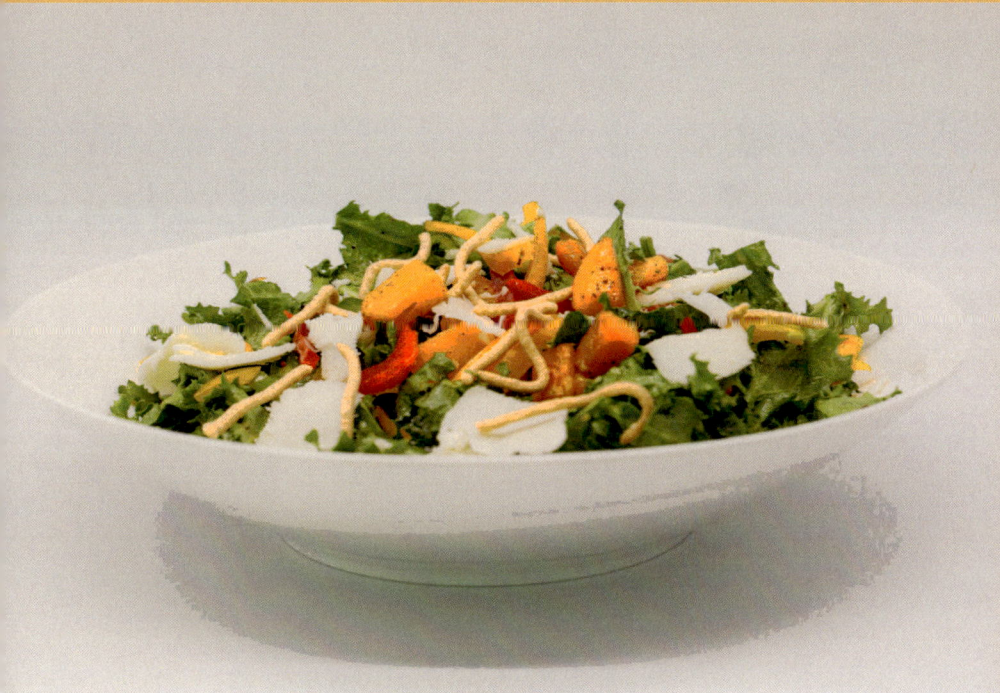

Directions

1 In a small frying pan, heat olive oil and add butternut, sauté for 5 minutes, set aside to cool down.

2 In a large bowl, add the spring mix. add bell peppers, and butternut squash. Top with Chow Mein noodles or crushed walnut, and feta or goat cheese.

3 Add chipotle vinaigrette and toss the salad a couple of times for great saturation.
Serve the salad as a side dish or a meal on its own.

Kale Apple Salad with Dates

25 minutes and 6 servings

Ingredients

½ tsp kosher salt
2 tbsp balsamic vinegar
½ tsp black pepper
4 cups chopped (stems removed)
1/2 cup dates shopped
½ pink lady apple cut in julienne
¼ cup asiago cheese cut in small thin pieces
2 tbsp extra virgin olive oil
1 tsp dried parsley

Go green, live more! This salad is tasty and crunchy It can also be topped with toasted walnut.

Bold and green, kale is a nutrient dense food. It's an excellent source of vitamins and anti-oxidants.

Directions

1 In a big salad bowl, whisk together olive oil, balsamic vinegar, salt, and dried parsley. Add the kale, toss to coat, massage and set it aside to rest for 8 -10 minutes

2 After 8 -10 minutes passed, add dates, apple, and cheese to the kale. Season with black pepper, toss a couple times and enjoy!

Lovely Romaine Chicken Wraps

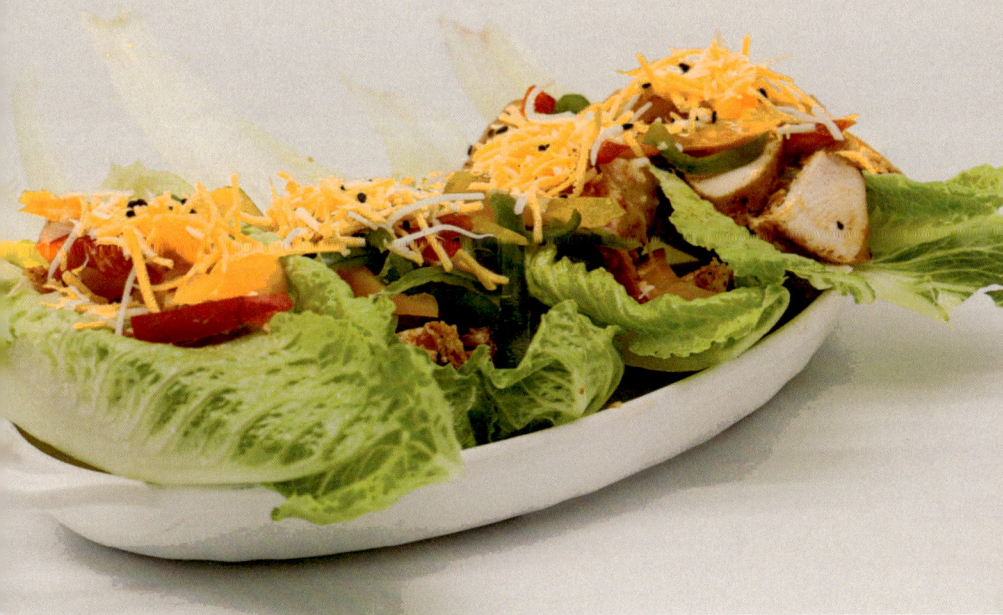

Ingredients

2 medium cut boneless
   chicken breasts
3 tbsp classic Rub Sause
1 bag romaine lettuce
(pull leaves apart)
½ cup shredded cheese
1 tsp caraway seed (optional)
1 cup sliced mix bell peppers
   (yellow, red, and green)
2 tbsp olive oil

Directions

1   Under cold water, rinse the chicken and cut into small
size cubes. Transfer the chicken to a clean bowl.

2   Add the classic rub and marinate for 10
minutes. Meanwhile, lay the romaine lettuce
flat on a tray.

3   In a medium frying pan, heat the oil, add the
chicken and sauté' thoroughly for 8-10
minutes or until brown. Remove the chicken
and set aside.

4   Add 4 to 6 cubes of chicken to all the lettuce, add
bell peppers, and sprinkle cheese over them
Top the wraps with caraway seed for extra
crunchiness and enjoy.

*These wraps are amazing and
flavorful!
They are a great substitute for
bread on low carb days.
This is a time efficient dish
that you and your family will
enjoy on busy days.
You can also use sesame seed
or hempseed for topping.*

*Romaine lettuce is a power
house, rich in minerals and
vitamins.*

Artichoke Panache'

10 minutes • Makes 4 servings

Ingredients

1 cup grape tomatoes
2 cups spring mix salad
1 can artichoke
2 tbsp feta cheese
¼ cup shaved mozzarella
1 tbsp rice vinegar
1 tbsp sesame oil
1 tsp minced ginger
1 tbsp tamarin sauce
1 tsp black pepper

Directions

1 In a small jar, shake together the tamarin sauce, rice vinegar, sesame oil, minced ginger and black pepper.

2 In a small bowl, add grape tomatoes, artichoke, shaved mozzarella: pour the dressing and toss it until all saturated.

3 In a big bowl, arrange the springs first, then add grape tomato mix, top with feta cheese and enjoy!

Tip: For this flavorful and colorful artichoke panache' use only the very freshest, grape tomatoes and spring m

Artichoke are rich in antioxidants an low in fat. They are high in fiber and loaded with vitamins and minerals.

Glazed Salmon with Coconut Milk Served with Green Garden Salad

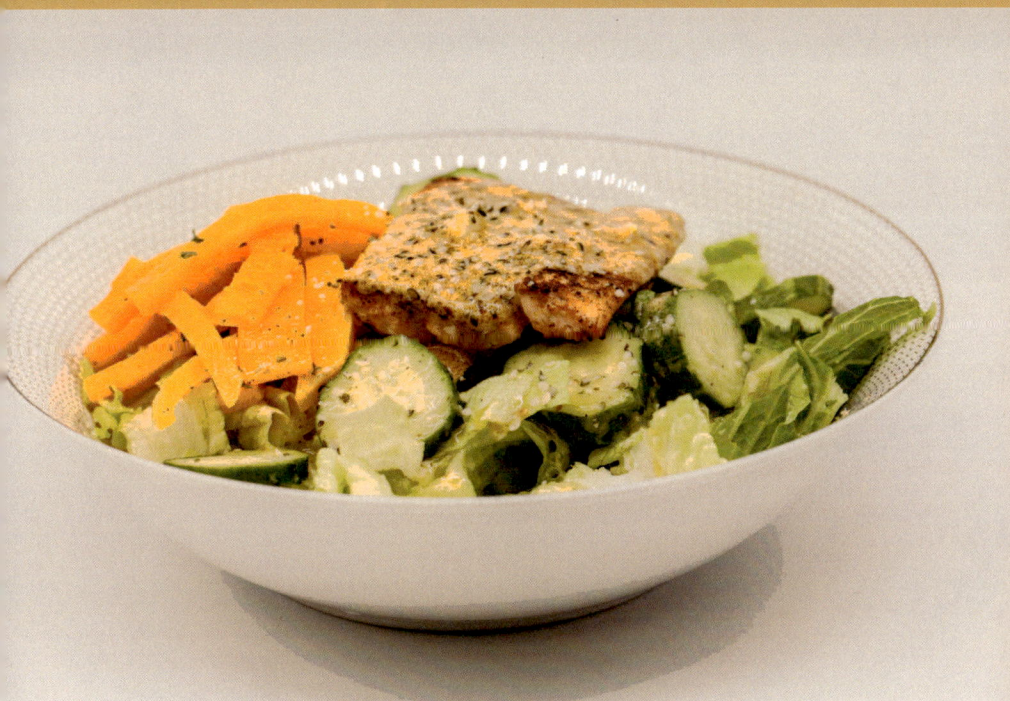

1 serving and 15-20 minutes

Ingredients

1 salmon fillet
½ cup les graines de vie's chipotle marinade sauce
1 cup coconut milk
1 tbsp olive oil
2 tbsp Irish butter
2 cups spring mix (lettuce)
1 medium cucumber
½ cup cherry tomatoes
¼ cup curry powder
Les graines de vie's honey lemon dijon vinaigrette
2 tbsp black caraway seeds

Directions

1 Rinse the fillet under cold water and place it in a bowl. Add the marinade and let it rest for 10-15 minutes.
After 10 minutes, in a skillet, add butter and olive oil on a medium low heat and place the fillet. Sauté it until golden brown and set aside.

2 In the same skillet, add coconut milk, curry powder and les graines de vie's marinade and let it cook for 5 minutes.
Pour coconut curry sauce over the fish and set aside.

3 In another large bowl, add mixed lettuce, cucumber, cherry tomatoes, les graines de vie's honey lemon dijon vinaigrette and mix well until all elements are well incorporated.
Serve the salad with the fillet salmon and top it with black caraway seeds and enjoy!

For this dish to have more servings, adjust the quantity of the ingredients, especially fish fillet and lettuce. Salmon is rich in omega-3 Fatty Acids, and a great source of protein, loaded with selenium

Healthy and Comfort Soups

Made with fresh ingredients

Soups are very simple to make but yet delicious and full of nutrients. They can be made with various ingredients such as vegetables, legumes, whole grains, broth and pair with protein or seafood.

Mellow Sweet Potato Soup

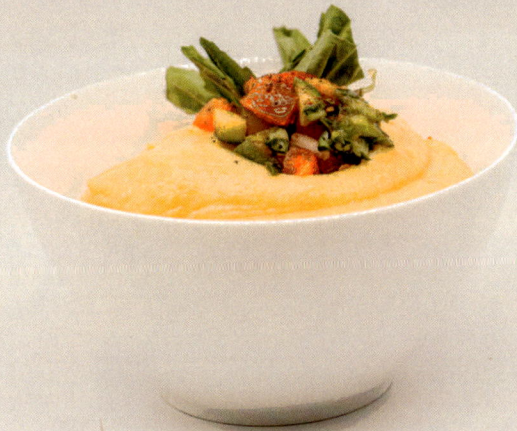

25 minutes and 5 servings

Ingredients

1 medium peeled and cubed sweet potato (orange)
2 small red bliss peeled and cubed potatoes
2 medium sweet potatoes (Japanese Yam) cubed
1 medium Yukon gold potato
2 tbsp sour cream/coconut cream
1 tsp nutmeg
2 cups potato stock (from boiling potatoes)
1 tsp Irish butter
1 cup vegetable or chicken stock
2 tbsp salsa de fresca

Directions

1   Turn the burner on high heat. In a big pot, add the potatoes, add plenty of water to cover the tops of the potatoes to ensure even cooking. Cover the lid and cook the potatoes for 15 minutes or until soft.
In a colander, drain the water from potatoes and set aside in another bowl for blending.

2   Transfer the cooked potatoes to a big mixing bowl. Add butter, nutmeg, sour cream, then potato water.
With a hand blender or immersion, blend the potatoes to a light and creamy consistency.
Pause for 30 seconds and check the texture. At this point, it should be thick and fluffy.

3   Slowly add the vegetable or chicken stock to the mixture and blend a couple of times for the final touch.
Serve the soup in a clean bowl, top it with salsa de fresca (Pico de galo) garnish with fresh mint leaves. Enjoy!

Potatoes are staple foods in many cultures. They are packed with fiber and rich in vitamin C and B6.

Golden and bold, this soup stands out as excellent and flavorsome.
Try it for yourself!

Golden Pumpkin Soup

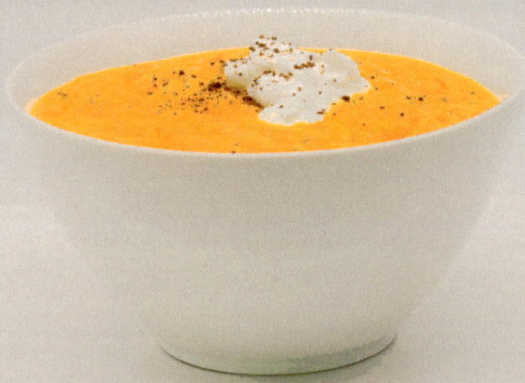

Ingredients

1 cup of mirepoix
(onion, celery and carrot)
1 tsp grated ginger
3 cups pumpkin puree
2 cups vegetable stock
1 tsp Indian salt
1 can coconut milk
1 tsp curry powder
2 tbs coconut oil
1tsp cinnamon(optional)
2 tbsp sour cream

Directions

1 Over medium heat, heat coconut oil in a sauce pan, add ginger and cook for one minute. Then add curry powder and give it a good stir and let it cook for one more minute or until the aroma is wafting from the pan.

2 Add the vegetable stock and coconut milk. Bring to a boil, reduce the heat to medium-low and let the mixer simmer for 5 minutes.

3 In a blender or food processor, add the puree, the mixer, Indian salt, cinnamon, mirepoix and blend to a smooth consistency.

This soup is filling and comforting. It can also be vegan by omitting the sour cream, just use coconut butter or cream instead.

4 Serve the soup in a bowl, top it with sour cream and a dash of cinnamon. Enjoy with gladness!

Togolese Ragoút de Pomme de Terre "aka" Potato Ragout

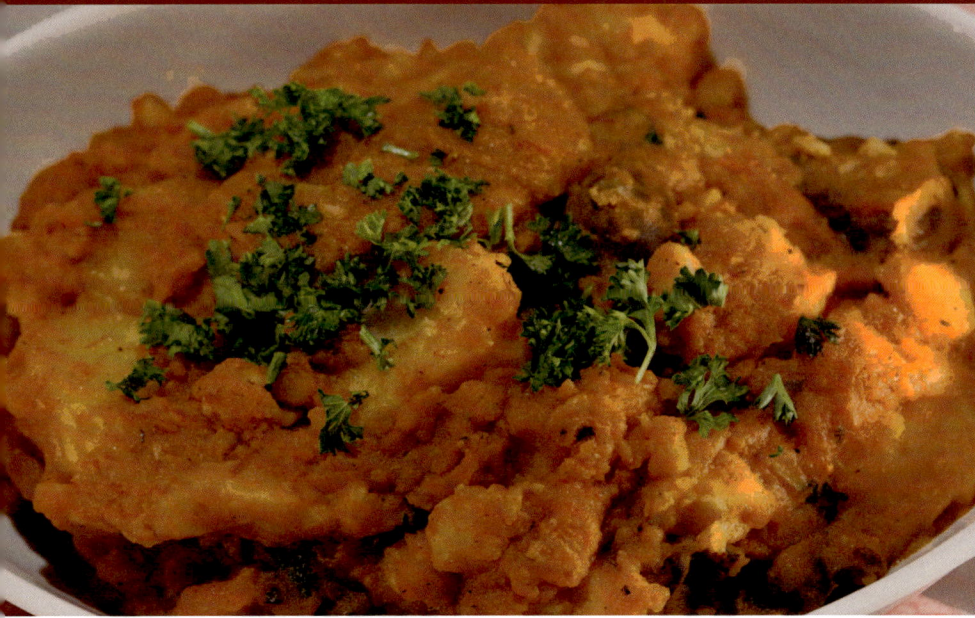

35 minutes and 8 servings

Ingredients

5 large Yukon gold potatoes peeled & quartered
I cup mirepoix (onion, celery and carrot) Optional see page
2 tbsp tomato paste
3 cups marinara tomato sauce or fresh tomato
1 cup dried tomato (optional)
¼ coconut oil or avocado

1 tsp kosher salt
2 tbsp bouillon seasoning or stock
2 bunches fresh parsley
2 cloves garlic minced
1 cup red onion diced
1 pound ½ cubed beef soup cut
2 tsp smoked paprika
1 tsp oregano
3 to 4 cups water

Ragout is one of my childhood favorite foods. The steps are easy. It can also be done in a crock-pot by adding all ingredients at once and slow-cooked.

Directions

1 In a large saucepan, add coconut oil over medium heat, garlic and sauté' for 1 minute. Add cubed beef, stock and sauté for 3 minutes until slightly brown.

2 Add tomato paste, stir often to prevent burning at the bottom of the pan for about 4 minutes. Add tomato sauce, mirepoix, smoked paprika. Bring water to a boil.

3 Add potatoes, salt, oregano, onion. Give a good stir and cover the pan.

4 Cook the ragout for 15 minutes until potatoes are soft. Reduce heat and simmer for 5 minutes for a creamy consistency.

5 Serve the ragout warm, top with fresh parsley and enjoy! Don't forget to pat yourself on the back for your creativity!

Crackers & dips

Crunchy and loaded with fiber

Crackers are my go-to snacks. I love munching on crackers. One thing that was very hard for me to let go when I decided to eat healthier, was the salty cracker. Even though I knew they were no good for me, I'd still get some; then afterwards, I would have edema all over my ankles. One day I said enough of this. That's when I came up with Les Graines de Vie Healthy Crackers. They are delicious and packed with a ton of nutrients and fiber. They're also low sodium and filling. What else is needed in a cracker? If you like to snack, call it your new BCF (Best Cracker Forever). I hope it will satisfy your craving as it has mine.

Almond Parmesan Cheese Crackers

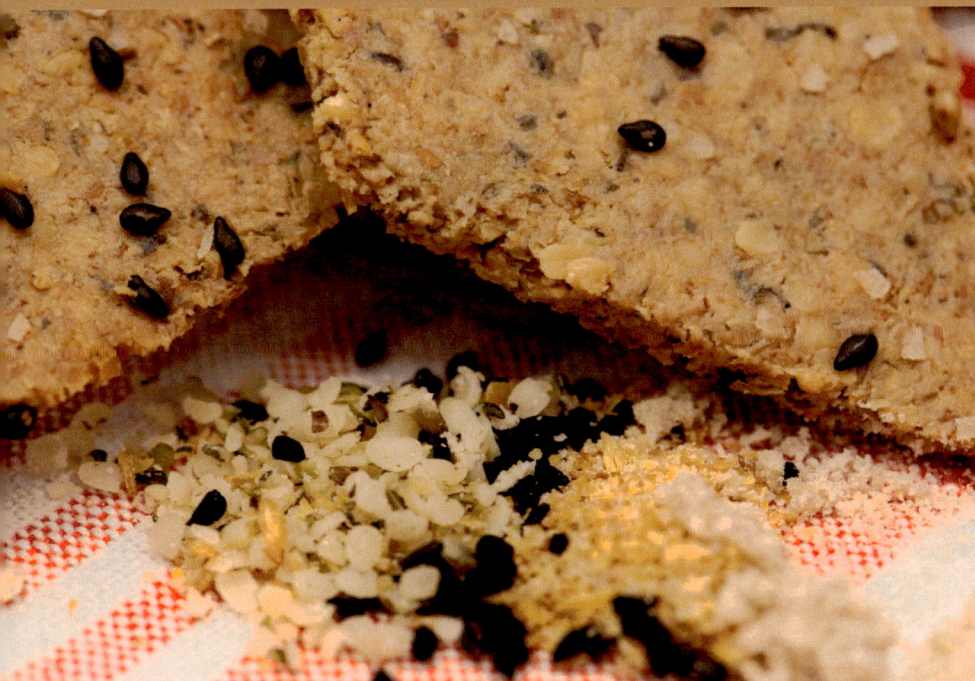

45 minutes 25 – 30 pieces or 6 servings

Ingredients

4 cups almond flour
2 cups parmesan cheese
1 cup flax seed meals
1 tsp kosher salt
1 tsp black peppers
½ smoked paprika
1 tsp garlic powder
1 tsp onion powder
2 tbs olive oil
1 cup of warm water

To make these crackers vegan, omit cheese. They are equally delicious!

Almonds are a source of healthy fats, protein, fiber, magnesium and Vitamin E.

Directions

1 In a medium bowl, combine all the elements and mix well until it is a firm consistent dough. Cover it up with a kitchen towel or plastic wrap for 10 minutes, for the dough to rest.

2 On wide square parchment paper, add the dough and cover with plastic wrap or with another parchment paper.

3 Flatten the dough to 1 inch thick and cut it in squares.

4 Turn the oven to 350 degrees Fahrenheit and lay the crackers on a baking sheet, you can add a dash of salt or black pepper for topping and bake it for 12-15 minutes.

5 After they are done, let them cool off and enjoy! Pat yourself on the back and smile!

Quinoa Crackers

30 minutes and 18 pieces, about 3 servings

Ingredients

1 cooked Quinoa
1 tsp Marjoram
3 tbsp chia seeds
1 tbsp olive oil
½ tsp kosher salt
1 tsp minced onion
½ cup brown rice flour
2 to 3 tbsp warm water
2 tbsp flax seed mea

Directions

1 Preheat the oven to 350 degree F. In a clean bowl, add Quinoa, marjoram, chia seeds, oil, salt, onion, brown rice, flax seed and water.

2 With a spatula, stir all the ingredients into a nice dough. Hands are better for shaping the dough. It should be a little firm and not sticky. Cover it up with kitchen tower or plastic wrap for 10 Minutes for the dough to rest.

3 On wide square parchment paper, add the dough and cover with plastic wrap or with another parchment paper. Flatten the dough to 1 inch thick and cut it in squares. Lay the crackers on a baking sheet, you can add a dash of salt or black pepper for topping and bake it for 12-15 Minutes.

4 After they are done, let them cool off and enjoy! Pat yourself on the back and smile!

These quinoa crackers are very filling and a great healthy snack

Quinoa is loaded with protein, rich in iron, high in magnesium and mostly low in calories. Great substitute for white rice! Quinoa is a whole grain.

Sunflower Seed Flour & Hempseed Crackers

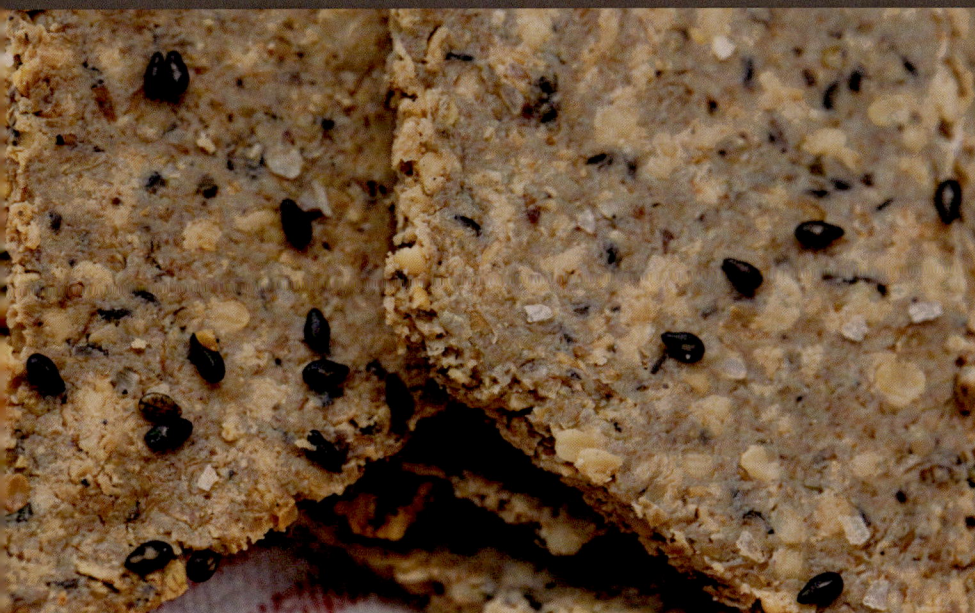

45 minutes 18 -20 pieces/ 4 servings

Ingredients

2 cups sunflower seed flour
1 cup hempseed
½ cup flax meal
½ rosemary
½ garlic powder
2 tbsp grape seed oil
1 tbsp black sesame seed
¼ warm water one drop at the time

These crackers are totally vegan and delicious. The hempseed give the cracker a buttery taste, yet crunchy.

Sunflower seeds are an excellent source of B complex Vitamins

Directions

1 1.In a big mixing bowl, add sunflower seed flour, hempseed, flax meal, rosemary, garlic powder, oil, and warm water.

2 Mix well until a firm consistency. Cover dough with a kitchen towel or plastic wrap for 10 minutes for the dough to rest.

3 On wide square parchment paper, add the dough and cover with plastic wrap or with another parchment paper. Flatten the dough to I inch thick and cut it in squares.

4 Turn the oven to 350 degrees Fahrenheit and lay the crackers on a baking sheet, you can add a dash of salt or black pepper for topping and bake it for 12-15 minutes.

5 After they are done, let them cool off and enjoy! Pat yourself on the back and smile!

Chickpea Dip "aka" Hummus

10 minutes and multiple servin

Ingredients

1 ½ cup cooked chickpeas
   (one can)
1 tbsp Tahini
(sesame seed butter)
2 tbsp olive oil
1 tbsp smoked paprika
2 cloves garlic
1 tsp chipotle spice
½ tsp salt (optional)
1 tsp black pepper
¼ cup warm water

Chickpea dip is a staple food in the Middle East and other parts of the World. Freshly homemade, it lasts 3 to 4 days in the fridge.

Chickpeas are high in protein and are a great substitute for meat for vegan and vegetarian diets. In addition, they are rich in vitamins, minerals and fiber.

Directions

1 In a blender or food processor, add chickpea, tahini, 1 tbsp olive oil, smoked paprika, garlic, black pepper, salt, warm water and blend the ingredients to a creamy consistency.

2 Store hummus into an air tight glass for future use. Or pour it into a bowl, dash the rest of the olive oil with a sprinkle of chipotle is staple food in middle East and enjoy it with some good homemade crackers.

Butter Beans Guacamole

10 minutes and multiple servings

Ingredients

1 bag frozen butter beans
(lima beans)
2 cups curly parsley shopped
2 tbsp sour cream or coconut cream
1 tsp Indian black salt or kosher salt
½ cup olive oil divided in half
(1/4 cup)
Pinch pepper flake
(optional for a kick)
1 tsp black pepper
1 tsp dried parsley
1 tsp garlic powder (optional)
1 tsp dry minced onion (optional)
1 cup water

Directions

1   In a colander, rinse the butter beans under cold water for 1 minute. In a small heated sauce pan, add the beans, ¼ olive oil, dried parsley, pepper flakes, salt, garlic powder, minced onion, and water. Cook the mixture for 15 minutes or until beans are tender and mushy.

2   Reduce to heat and simmer the beans to absorb the liquid for 2 more minutes. In a food processor, add fresh parsley, water and pulse a couple of times. Add butter beans, ¼ cup left over olive oil, sour cream or coconut cream. Blend the butter beans to a creamy consistency (open the blender and stir a couple of times).

3   Pour butter beans into a bowl and enjoy with your favorite crackers and chips on game days

At my lab ,"aka" kitchen, every dish has a story. This one goes like this: Once upon a time, avocados became "Diamonds" in the land of South Korea. So I decided to make my kid's favorite dip, a healthier reality. I found out, my independent variables and dependent variables supported my hypothesis. Voila, guacamole was born that day

Lunches Under 30 Minutes

Nutrient Dense

Eating a healthy lunch is crucial for many reasons. Food strengthens us and boost our immune system. When eating a healthy lunch, we are able to avoid any unnecessary mid-afternoon snacks that are loaded with salt or sugar.

Delightful Zucchini Tots

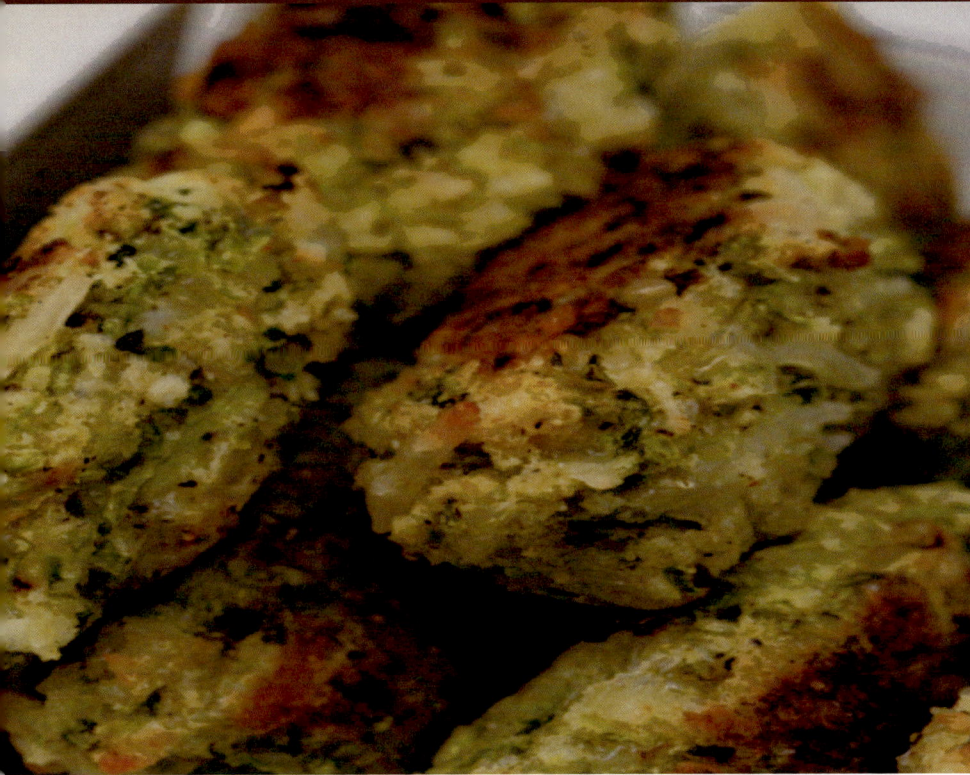

These zucchini tots are breath taking, crunchy, yet soft on the inside. If you opt for a vegan choice, omit cheese and eggs. Instead, use flaxseed meal for binding. This recipe yields 20 servings and takes 30-35 minutes to prepare.

Ingredients

4 cups panko breadcrumbs
3 cups parmesan cheese
6 eggs
2 tsp garlic powder
2 tsp black pepper
1 tbsp kosher salt,
1 tbsp onion powder
16 medium-sized zucchini
1 tbsp Irish butter (grease baking sheet)

Incorporating zucchini is a healthy way to add veggies into your diet and your family's diet. Zucchini are saturated with water. They have essential nutrients and vitamins such as A and C, potassium, fiber, and folate.

Directions

1. Preheat oven to 400°F (200°C.)
2. Shred the zucchini in a food processor, sprinkle salt and give a quick massage.
3. Allow zucchini to sit for 10-15 minutes as the salt draws out moisture.
4. Pour zucchini onto a clean dish towel, or a cheese cloth and drain all the water out.
5. Pour the zucchini back into your bowl and add breadcrumbs, parmesan cheese, eggs, garlic powder, onion powder and pepper. Mix until well-blended.
6. Take a tablespoon of the mixture and roll it into a tot, until all completed.
7. Put the tots on a greased baking sheet and place in the oven for 20-25 minutes or until tots are crunchy and lightly brown. Serve warm and enjoy!

Seaweed Seasoned Brown Rice

9 servings and 40 minutes

Ingredients

1 bag brown rice (2 cups)
1 pack seasoning seaweed
2 tbsp séaseme seed oil
Chipotle seasoning
1 cup mixed bell peppers
  (red, yellow and green)

Directions

1 In a large bowl, rinse brown rice under cold water. Cover the rice with warm water to the tops and soak for 2 hours or overnight.

2 Turn the stove to medium heat in a sauce pan rinse rice again about 3 times add 6 cups of water and bring to a boil for 30 minutes or until all water is absorbed. Reduce the heat and simmer for 5 more minutes for a sticky texture for this dish.

3 In a large bowl, add cooked brown rice, oil, chipotle, seasoned seaweed, mixed bell peppers and mix well until all ingredients are incorporated.

4 Shape the rice into a ball by using a small bowl or a big ice cream scooper.
Serve along with baked fish, sautéed asparagus, and enjoy!

This sticky rice is delicious and wholesome. If you don't like brown rice, you will fall in love and incorporate it into your diet.
Always rinse well the grains before cooking. Whole grains like brown rice should be soaked in order to ease digestion and also release more nutrients.

Brown rice is a whole grain rich in fiber, it promotes fullness. It 's a " low-glycemic index " food

Eggplant Mushroom Stew

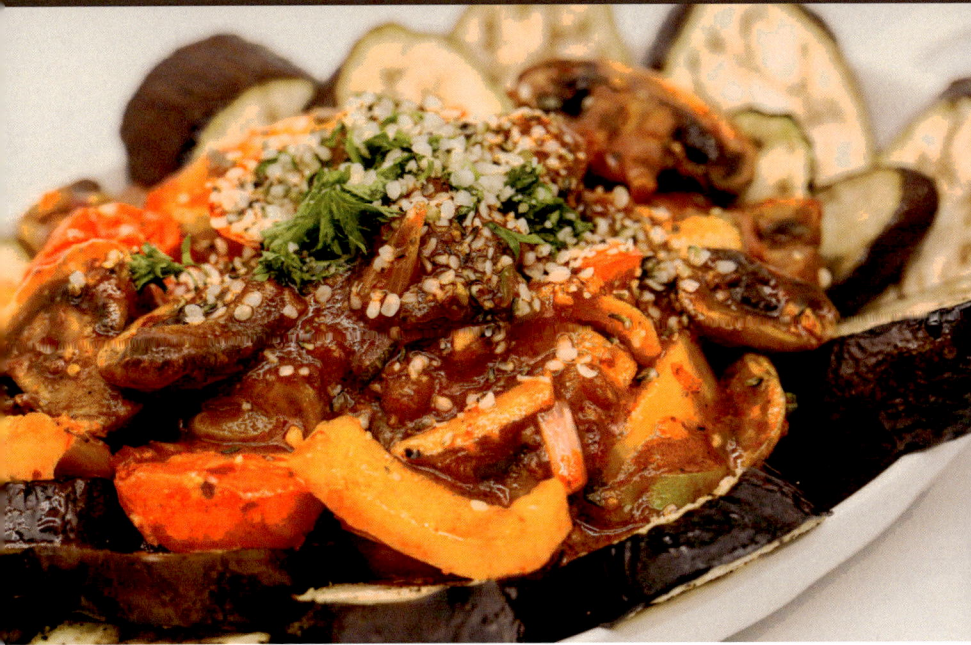

Ingredients

2 tablespoon Thai chili Garlic
  sauce
¼ cup of coconut oil or olive
  oil
3 medium to large eggplant
4 garlic gloves
¼ slice medium onion
1tsp kosher salt
1 tsp tamarin sauce
½ tsp black pepper
3 cups Shiitake Mushroom
  (based on family size)
1 tsp Les Graines de vie's
  Bouillon (optional} or
  stock
2 tbsp shopped parsley
1 tsp hempseed (optional)

*Eggplant are loaded with
high fiber, rich in nutrients
such as vitamin C, K, B6,
niacin, folic acid and more…
yet low-calories.*

Directions

1 Turn the oven to 350 C. Cut the eggplant in pieces
and place in a bowl. Dash olive oil and salt, black
pepper and toss a couple of times. On a baking
sheet, transfer the eggplant and bake for 10-15
minutes. In a mortar/pestle crush garlic and onion.
In a medium heated work, add coconut oil/olive oil.
Sauté' the crushed garlic-onion for 1 minute.
Add mushroom and sauté' for 4 minutes.

2 Take them out and add 2 tbsp Thai garlic chili sauce
to the work, let it cook for 3 Minutes.
Add Les Grained de vie's bouillon seasoning or
stock of your choice to the sauce, then pour the
mushroom over it and give a good mix.

3 Taste the sauce and adjust the flavor to your likeness.
Lay the eggplant in a plate next to each other to form
a round shape by closing the center. Pour the sauce
in the center until you reach the periphery of the
plate. Serve the sauce along with any whole grains.
Dash parsley, hempseed and enjoy!

Savory Vegetable Medley

20 minutes and 6 servings

Ingredients

1 bag frozen mixed vegetables
1 medium quartered sweet
  potato
1 medium white golden potato
  quartered
1 cup of cubed butternut squash
1 tsp salt
1 black pepper
2 tbsp Irish butter or ghee
  butter
1 clove garlic grated
1 tbsp parmesan cheese to top
  (optional)

Directions

1 In a large colander, rinse the vegetable mix under cold water and set aside.

2 Turn the burner on medium heat. In a sauce pan, add the potato and plenty of water to cover the tops of potatoes. Bring to a boil for 8 minutes by about halfway cooked. Drain the water and set aside.

3 In large work, add butter and garlic, sauté for 30 seconds, pour the vegetable mix and potatoes. Dash salt, black pepper and toss a few times. Sauté the medley for 5 more minutes. Reduce heat and simmer for another 30 seconds. Serve the medley warm and enjoy it as side dish

This medley can also be a complete meal if paired with a protein.
This is my kid's favorite, because it actually tastes delicious.
The savory flavor is unforgettable.

Oregano-Garlic Roasted Mixed Potatoes

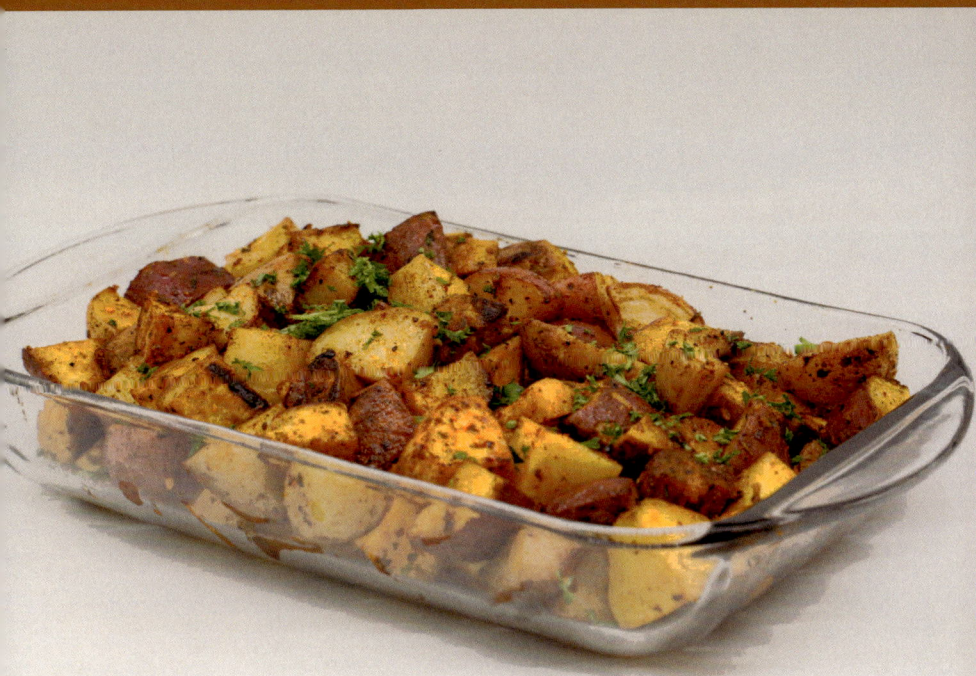

50 minutes regular way

(pre-boiled 25 minutes) 6 servings

Ingredients

1 large sweet potato (orange)
2 medium red bliss potatoes
2 large sweet potatoes
   (Japanese Yam)
2 medium Yukon gold
   potatoes
3 tbsp olive oil
1 tsp kosher salt
2 tbsp chipotle & roasted
   garlic
1 tbsp garlic powder or
   minced
1 tsp dried parsley
1 tbsp minced fresh parsley
   (garnish)
1 tbsp oregano
1 tbsp smoked paprika
1 tsp black pepper

To reduce the baking time of these potatoes in half, after you cut them quarterly, boil them first for 5-10 minutes, then roast.
Now the baking time will be less, but also they will be crispy and delicious. That is the trick!

Directions

1 Preheat the oven to 400 degrees F or 205 degrees C. In large mixing bowl, wash the potatoes well and remove any residue or soil. Cut the potatoes in quarters, place them in the bowl and set aside.

2 In a small bowl, add olive oil, salt, chipotle, parsley, oregano, smoked paprika, minced garlic and give a good stir. Dress the potatoes with the mixer and toss for a couple of times until the potatoes are well coated. Transfer the potatoes to the baking sheet and disperse them evenly.

3 Dash black pepper all over the potatoes. Roast potatoes for 40-55 minutes until golden brown (raw potatoes). Roast for 25 minutes (preboil) potatoes until golden and crispy. Turn the potatoes over twice for a uniform browning.
Take potatoes from oven. Serve them hot and top with fresh parsley. Enjoy your creativity!

Rotini a La Sauce De Tomate

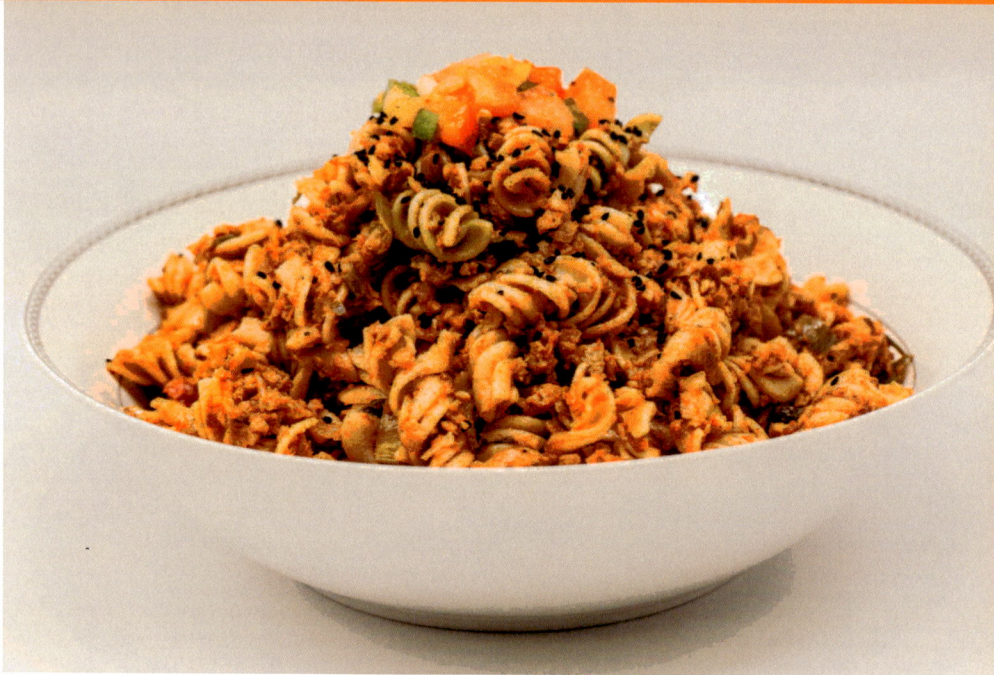

Ingredients

1 box rotini pasta (whole-wheat is more nutritious)
1 cup high protein TVP---- Textured Vegetable Protein (dried Soy)
3 cups marinara tomato sauce
¼ cup olive oil
½ diced onion
1 tsp kosher salt
1 tsp vegetable bouillon powder
2 garlic cloves
1 tsp grated ginger
1 tsp caraway seed (optional)

This dish is 100 % vegan and delicious
for meatless meals.
For gluten sensitivity, opt for gluten free pasta instead of whole-wheat.

Directions

1 Bring 4-6 quarts of water to a boil.
Add salt and pasta to boiling water. Boil the pasta for 6-7 minutes. Drain well and set aside.

2 In a large heated work, add oil, ginger, garlic and sauté for 1 minute.
Add the dried soy (protein textured) and cook for 3 minutes, then add marinara tomato sauce. Reduce the heat to medium to simmer for 5 minutes.

3 Add the vegetable bouillon, salt, onion and stir well. Taste the sauce and adjust the flavor if needed. Add the pasta and toss a couple of times until all is well saturated. Cook the pasta for another 2 minutes. Serve the pasta hot, top it with caraway seed and enjoy!

Delightful Greens & Fish

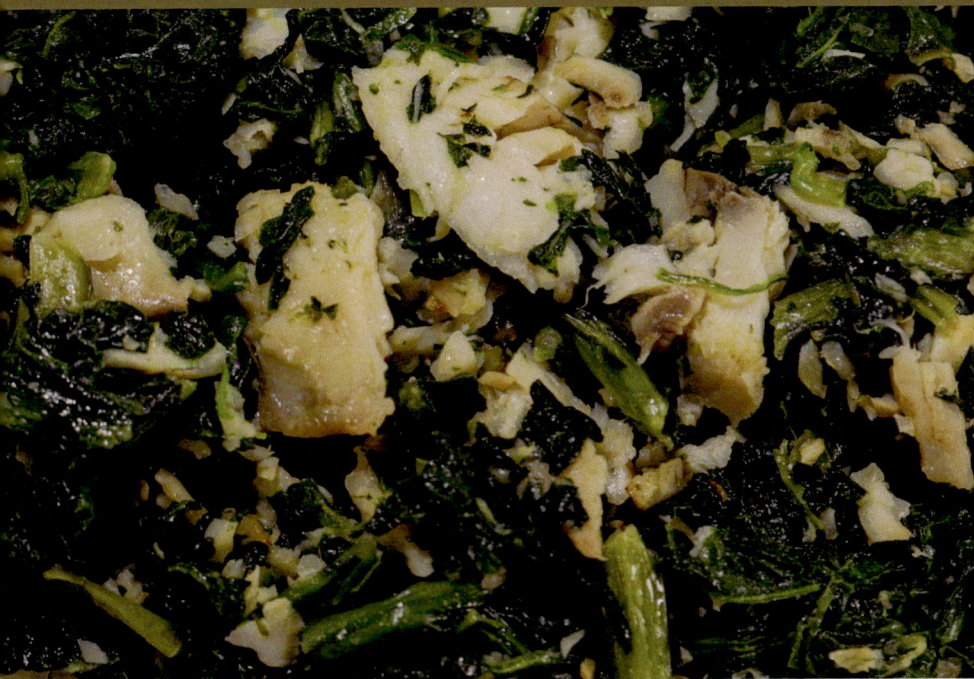

10 minutes and 3 of servings

Ingredients

6 cod fillets or tilapia
3 cups frozen spinach
3 cups frozen collard greens
   or turnip
3 gloves garlic chopped
2 tbsp LGDV's bouillon
   seasoning or any
   seasoning of your choice.
1 tsp dried cilantro
1 tsp hot pepper powder
   (optional)
¼ cup chopped red onion
2 tbsp olive oil
1 tsp kosher salt
2 tbsp LGDV's rub

This dish is a great way to combine greens and sea food.

This dish is a great way to combine greens and sea food. Fish are an *excellent* source of protein and minerals.

Directions

1 Rinse the fillets under cold water and place them in a bowl. Add LGDV's rub, garlic, dried cilantro and set aside.

2 In a strainer, rinse the greens and press down several times for extra water, or squeeze the water out with your hands in small batches.

3 Turn the burner to medium heat, add olive oil, garlic, and the tilapia fillet. Sauté' for 5 minutes until it becomes opaque, and flaky.

4 Add the greens, hot pepper, chopped onion, bouillon seasoning and salt. Give it a good stir until the greens are well saturated.

5 Cook the mix for another 2 minutes, taste it and adjust the flavor if needed. Serve the greens with any grain of your choice. It can also be a side dish to any sea food main course.

Golden Cauliflower & Corn Rice

Cauliflower rice is adaptable to many ways of cooking. One Caution: It doesn't like extra water. To make it successful, pull out all the moisture.

Ingredients

1 medium cauliflower head
2 tbsp rub sauce (see pg..) or Thai chili
½ cup corn kernel
¼ cup diced red onion
½ cup mixed bell peppers (yellow, green, red)
Pinch of 3 in 1 (black pepper, salt, & garlic)
1 tbsp coconut oil

Directions

1. Rinse the cauliflower head and add to a food processor or blinder, shredded to a fine rice like shape

2. Soak the shredded cauliflower in water for 15 minutes.

3. After, pour cauliflower rice onto a clean dish towel or a cheese cloth and drain all the water out.

4. In a medium heat, over a large work, add coconut oil, rub sauce, diced onion, and cook for 2 minutes.

5. Add cauliflower rice, corn kernel, mixed bell peppers and toss a couple times.

6. Reduce the heat to simmer for 2 more minutes. Now dash 3 in 1 seasoning and stir one more time.

7. Remove the rice from the stove and serve warm with any protein of your choice.

Cauliflower is a cruciferous vegetable, rich in fiber and B vitamins. It's great for low carb diets and is a brain food because of Choline------a key ingredient

Lemon Garlic Butter Chicken

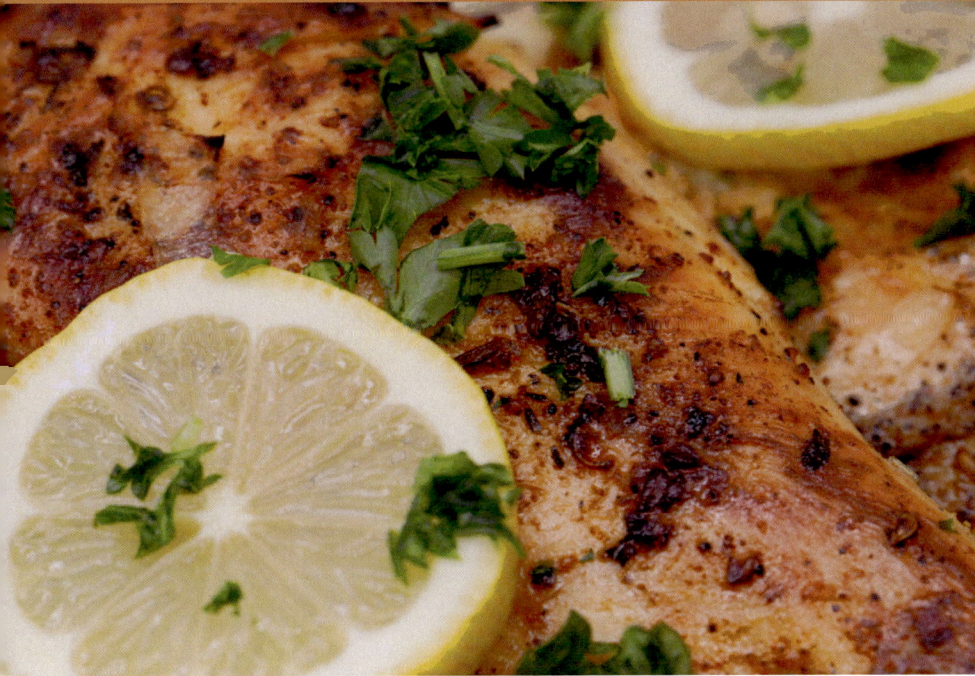

Ingredients

2 tbsp half & half or whole milk
6 pieces chicken breasts
1 tsp kosher salt
1 tsp black pepper
¼ cup Irish butter (half of stick)
2 tbsp olive oil
1 tsp chicken bouillon (optional)
3 cloves of garlic
1 tbsp diced white onion
3 cups chicken broth
2 tbsp lemon juice
1 tbsp chipotle seasoning
2 lemons slices (garnish)

Chicken is a lean meat and source of protein. Therefore, it's a great option for healthy eating.

These chicken breasts are heavenly!
To make the sauce even easier and creamier, make the roux first, then add other ingredients.
I have tried both and they are amazing. No compromise when it comes to taste!

Directions

1 Bag the chicken breasts in food grade plastic and pound them to thin cutlets. In a mixing bowl, season the chicken with salt, chipotle, black pepper, chicken bouillon and set aside.

2 In a medium heat fry pan, add olive oil, and sauté' chicken for 10 minutes until golden brown on both sides and set aside. Add butter, garlic and cook for 2 minutes until the aroma is strong on the same pan. Add the onion, lemon juice, and cook the mixture for another 3 minutes. Then add the milk slowly and whisk a couples of times for a lightly creamy texture.

3 Now add the chicken broth and give a good stir. Let the mixture simmer for 2 more minutes. Transfer the chicken to a baking sheet, poor the sauce over chicken beasts and bake for 15 minutes. Serve chicken warm, top with fresh parsley and lemon slices. Enjoy with one of your favorite grains or vegetables.

Bean Ragout with Italian Sausage

Ingredients

1 cup Italian grounded
  sausage
1 can pinto beans
1 can dark red kidney beans
  (Bush's)
1 cup butternut squash cubed
1 cup stock or bouillon
  seasoning
1 tsp dried parsley
3 minced garlic cloves
1 tsp tarragon dried or fresh
1 tbsp smoked paprika
1 tbsp 3 in one seasoning
  panache' (black pepper,
  red pepper flake and
  kosher salt)
½ cup marinade (tomato
  sauce)
¼ zucchini cubed
2 tbsp olive oil
½ cubed carrot

Beans are sources of protein, a dense food that controls appetite. They are filling and packed with great antioxidants. Great when paired with vegetables like squash and zucchini. What better way to eat healthy?!

Directions

In a clean calendar, drain and rinse the beans and put them a side. Turn the stove on medium-high heat.

In a medium sauce pan, add olive oil, garlic, carrot or Mirepoix (cooking base) Add the sausage, stirring for few seconds to break the sausage in small pieces and let it cook for 5 minutes or until brown.

Add the beans, butternut squash, dried parsley, seasoning panache', marinade, smoked paprika, tarragon, kosher salt, stock, cubed zucchini and cooked for 10 minutes.

Bring the heat to low setting and let the mixer cook for another 3 minutes until thicken.
Serve the ragout hot just like it is or use it as a side dish or a nacho deep like chili.
Now pat yourself on the back, smile and be proud!

Multi-Culture Healthy Foods

Nutrients Dense Breakfasts, Lunches, Dinners, and Snacks

Multi-culture Healthy foods are fascinating. Bold in colors and mesmerized your taste buds. I love all culture-foods.
Being a military family member, I am very fortunate to travel and stationed around the world. Food brings people together, If your are new in a country, the best way to make friend is to try locals food. You will be surprise How welcoming they local restaurant are.

Mediterranean Couscous Salad in Chipotle Vinaigrette

15 minutes and 3 servings

Ingredients

1 cup chopped red cabbage
1 cup chopped white cabbage
1 ½ cup cooked couscous
¼ medium onion finely sliced
3 tbsp chipotle dressing
¼ cup cubed zucchini
1 cup mixed bell peppers
  (yellow, orange, red and
  green)
3 to 5 pieces of snow peas
¼ cup red onion
1 bunch fresh parsley

This salad is very easy and delicious, the crunchiness of the cabbage gives this dish a scrumptious and fresh taste. Taste and see!

Cabbage is a smart carb to add into a diet. They help detoxify the body and are great for weight loss.

Directions

1   In a glass bowl, add couscous, cabbages (red and white), onion, zucchini, mixed bell peppers, snow peas and dressing.

2   Toss all the ingredients a few times until well combined.

3   Serve the salad topped with fresh parsley.

Senegalese Chicken Yassa

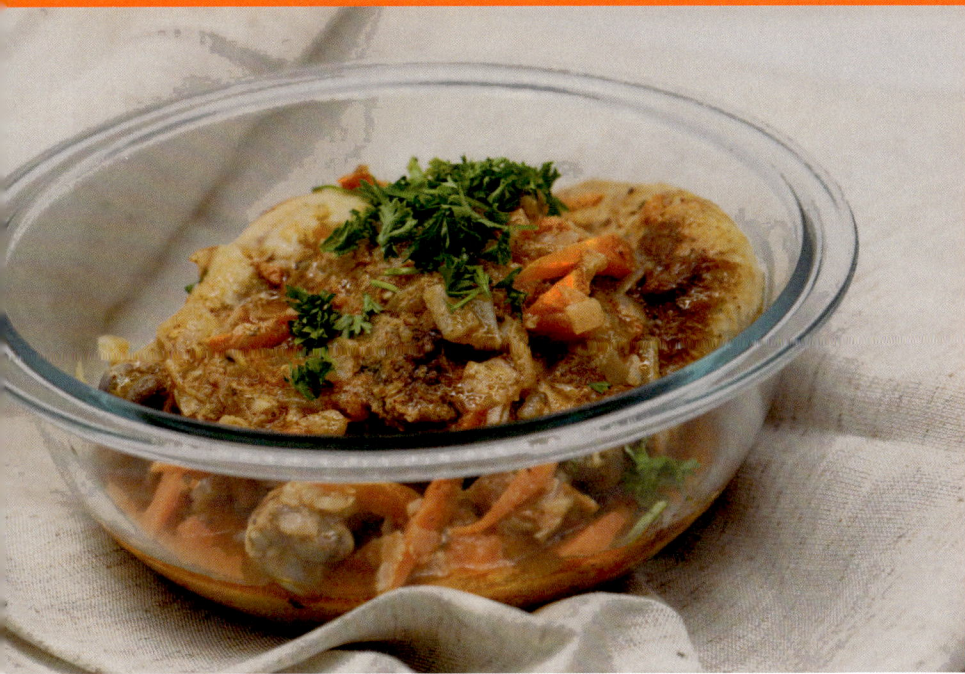

Ingredients

1 whole chicken, cut into
     pieces
1/2 cup freshly squeezed
     lemon juice
4 large onion, thinly
     sliced
5 tbsp olive oil
1 medium carrot sliced
2 tbsp Dijon mustard
1 tbsp Düsseldorf style
     mustard or yellow mustard
1 cup water
1 tsp kosher salt
2 tbsp Les Graines de vie's
     Bouillon seasoning or any
     seasoning of your choice
3 cloves of garlic minced
1 bunch fresh parsley
1 tsp smoked paprika
1 tsp cayenne pepper
1 tbsp tamarin sauce

*To make the process easy and
quick for this dish, marinate
the chicken overnight for a
strong flavor.*

Directions

1 In a large bowl, prepare marinade by mixing the lemon
juice, onions, salt, cayenne pepper, minced garlic, paprika,
Dijon mustard, onion, 1 tbsp olive oil, and tamarin sauce.
Place the chicken pieces in the marinade and saturate.
Cover the bowl with plastic wrap and allow the chicken to
marinate for at least 1 hour in the refrigerator.

2 In a heated large fried pan, add another 2 tbsp oil, sauté
the chicken pieces, lightly brown on both sides. Remove
the chicken and set aside. In a medium heated sauce pan,
add the remaining oil. Remove onions from the marinade
and add to the pan, cook the onion slowly until tender and
translucent.

3 Add the reserved marinade and cook for 3 minutes. When
the liquid is completely heated, add the chicken pieces,
carrots, water, Düsseldorf mustard, bouillon seasoning.
Bring the yassa slowly to simmer. Cover for about 30
minutes, or until the chicken is cooked through. Serve over
Couscous or brown rice and top the dish with fresh parsley
and enjoy!

61

Togolese (West Africa) Black Eyed-Pea Fritters

45 minutes 6 servings

Ingredients

1 pound dried black eye-peas
1 cup chopped shallots and
  onion
¼ cup chopped garlic
1 tsp kosher salt
1 tsp black pepper
1 tbsp hot pepper flake or
  habanero
1 tbsp Baking powder
4 cups grape seed oil or
  avocado (fried)
2 cups of water

Beans are a slow release of energy, and loaded with protein. They are nutrient dense foods and control appetite.

These bean fritters were my To-Go breakfast or snack when I was a little girl. Growing up in Togo (West Africa), beans were a staple food because they were cheap, and poor families could feel sustained for more hours in a day.

Directions

1. Rinse and soak the black eye-peas for 2 hours - 24 hours in advance. In a blender or food processor, combine all elements except baking powder and oil. Pulse a couple times and blend until you reach a smooth consistency.

2. In a big bowl, add the bean batter, baking powder, and whip with a whisk until it becomes fluffy. In a big frying pan, add grape seed oil or avocado oil to a medium high heat by 375 degrees.

3. Scoop the batter with an ice cream scooper and drop into the hot oil in little batches. Let them cook about 3-5 minutes turning once until golden brown.
Remove from hot oil with a slotted spoon, drain well with a paper towel and serve hot.

Golden Polenta

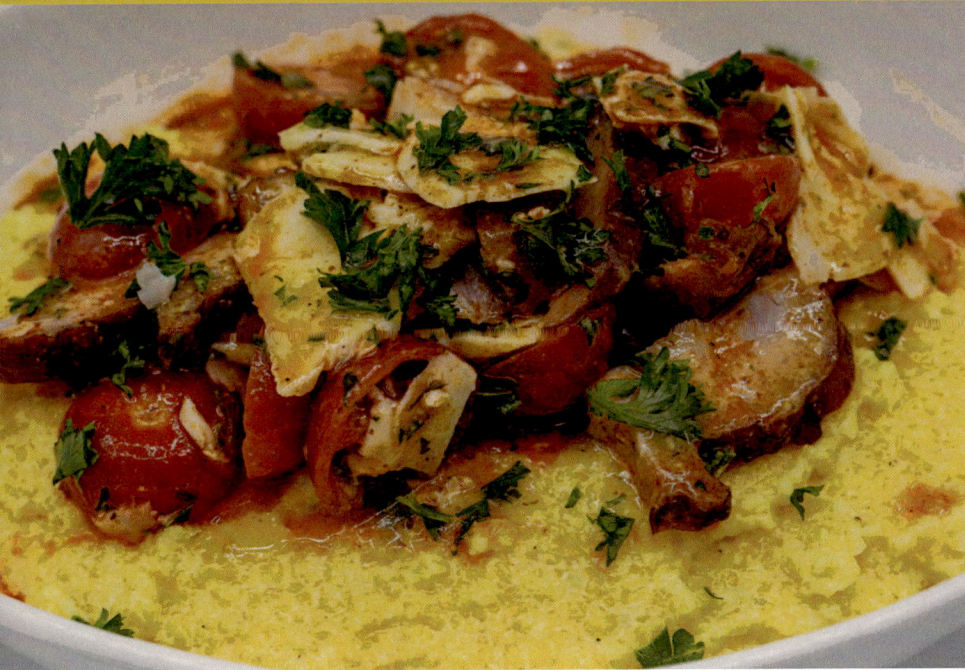

45 minutes and 4 servings

Ingredients

1 cup Polenta (coarse ground
    cornmeal)
3 ½ cups water
1 cup organic valley 100 %
    whole milk
2 tbsp ghee butter or Irish
1 tsp black pepper
1 tsp black Indian salt or
    kosher divided
1 cup cherry tomatoes
A couple slices of shredded
    mozzarella
1/4cup Parmigiano-Reggiano
1 bunch of curly parsley
    chopped
2 slices of bacon or smoked
    turkey (optional)
2 tbsp olive oil
1 tbsp lemon juice or
    balsamic vinegar

Directions

1. In a high heated medium sauce pan, bring water and salt to a boil. Slowly pour polenta into boiling water and whisk continuously to a smooth consistency without lumps.

2. Lower the heat and simmer polenta to a thick consistency, about seven minutes.
Whisk often, every 3 to 4 minutes and let it cook for a total of 25 minutes until creamy and soft in the taste.

3. Add butter, salt, milk. With a spatula, stir the polenta for taste and adjust the flavor, then turn the heat off. Add cheese, cover the pan and let it stand for 3 minutes. Meanwhile, in a little bowl, mix tomatoes, oil, smoked turkey slices, salt, black pepper, balsamic vinegar, mozzarella, Top polenta with the mixture, and garnish with fresh parsley.

Did you know that Polenta can also be made with millet, garbanzo beans or farro? The creativity is unlimited, so go ahead and explore.

To make it vegetarian, use mushroom instead of meat.

Mushroom Fettuccine with Pesto Sauce

Ingredients

1 cup shopped spinach
2 cups shopped curly parsley
1 cup Parmesan Romano shredded
1/ ½ cup Olive oil
5 Garlic cloves
1 ¼ cup divided in Grated Parmesan Romano
1 cup Vegetable stock or chicken stock
1 tsp Kosher salt
1 Fettuccini pasta pack
1 tsp Black pepper
½ cup diced onion
2 tbsp minced garlic
3 cups shiitake mushroom halves

Parsley is a powerful herb, rich in vitamin K which is necessary for bone health, calcium absorption and blood clotting. Parsley also reduces inflammation

For this dish, the mushroom ca be substituted with meat if desired.
The green bold color of this dis makes it so vivid and appetizing

Directions

1 In a big pot add water to a boil and cook the pasta according to the package instruction. You can also add some olive oil on the water to prevent stickiness of the pasta.

2 To make the pesto: In a food processor or blender, add parsley, garlic glove, olive oil (1 cup), salt and pulse a couple of time. Add 1 cup parmesan, stock and blend the mixer to a creamy sauce and set apart. Turn your stove to a medium heat, in a big work, add the ½ cup olive oil remaining, minced garlic, diced onion, black pepper, mushroom and sauté' for2 minutes, add the pesto to the pot and stir the sauce. Let it cook for another 5 minutes.

3 After 5 minutes passed, check the taste and adjust the flavor to your likeness. Add the pasta to the sauce and give it a good mix and let it cook for another 2 more minutes. Serve the pasta hot and sprinkle on top with the ¼ remaining parmesan Romano left and enjoy! Pat yourself on the back and smile.

Mushroom Coco Curry

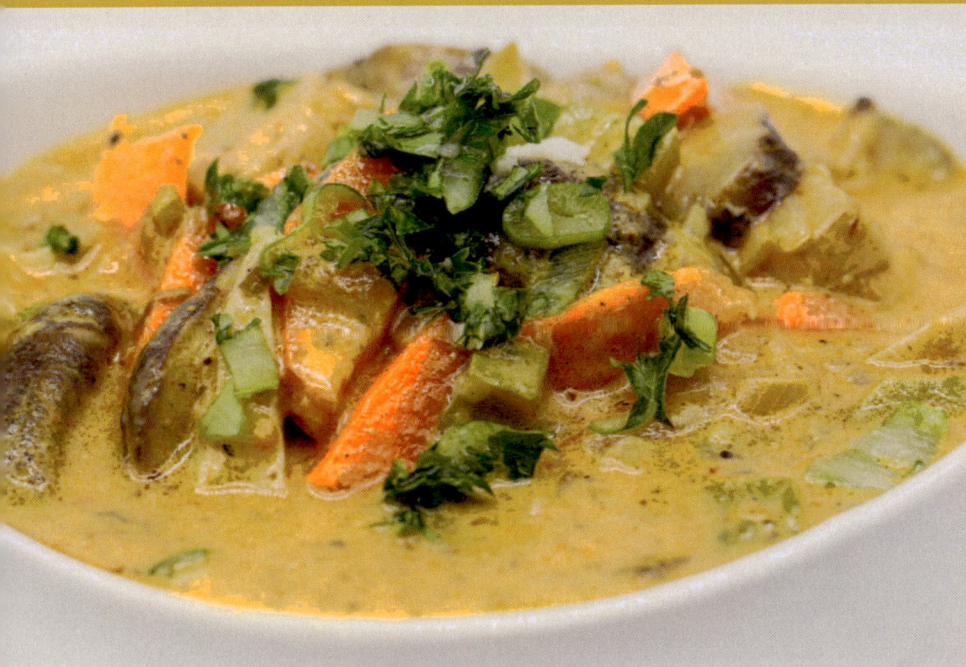

Ingredients

4 cups shiitake mushroom
1tbsp LGDV seasoning
   bouillon or stock
½ tsp kosher salt
1/2 sliced carrot
2 tbsp exotic curry powder
   (strong flavor)
1 tsp grated ginger
1 zucchini cubed
1 cup coconut milk
2 minced garlic cloves
1 tsp oregano
¼ cup fine chopped onion
1 tsp cayenne pepper
   (optional)
2 tbsp avocado oil
1 cup water

Directions

1. In a sauce pan, heat oil on medium –high, add garlic and ginger cook for 30 seconds.
Add onion, carrot, mushroom, water and let it cook for 3 minutes.

2. Add coconut milk, curry powder, cayenne peeper, oregano and stir well, cover the pan and let the mixer cook for another 5 minutes.

3. Add stock or bouillon powder, salt and reduce the heat low. Add cubed Zucchini and simmer the mixer for another 2 minutes
Serve the soup hot and enjoy.
The soup can be accompanied with any grain of your choice.

Mushroom coco curry is very versatile and can be made in one pot. This dish was created due to my longing to my home country . One day I just could not help it. I decided to go to my kitchen and make something, not too fancy yet a rich African exotic flavor .and Voila: Coco curry was born that day!

Togolese Crunchy Delicious Bread

15-20 buns 30 minutes

Ingredients

3 cups organic all purpose
  flour

3 larges eggs

¾ organic pure sugar or
coconut sugar

1/2 cup milk or water

4 tbsp Irish butter melted

2 tsp baking powder

½ tsp salt

5 – 7 cups grape-seed oil for
frying

1 tsp vanilla extra

3½ tsp nutmeg

*Great and easy snack for your sweet tooth once in a while. In some parts of Togo, people eat this bread for breakfast paired with a local porridge called "La Bouillie", that's French word for Porridge.

Directions

1   In a large bowl, combine, flour, sugar, salt, baking powder, nutmeg stir well and set aside.

2   In a small bowl, mix the wet ingredients by adding eggs, vanilla extra, melted butter, and water or milk.

3   Create a hole in center of the flour, pour wet ingredients into the hole, slowly stir the mixture in a circular motion until consistency is smooth, lightly sticky dough.

4   Heat the oil to 340-350 F on a medium work, use ice cream spoon to scoop out the mixture in a ball shape or your fingers.

5   Drop the balls into the oil and cook both sides for 3-4 minutes. Remove balls and drain the oil with paper towel.
Serve the crunchy bread hot and enjoy!

Togolese Peanut Butter Stew with Collard Greens

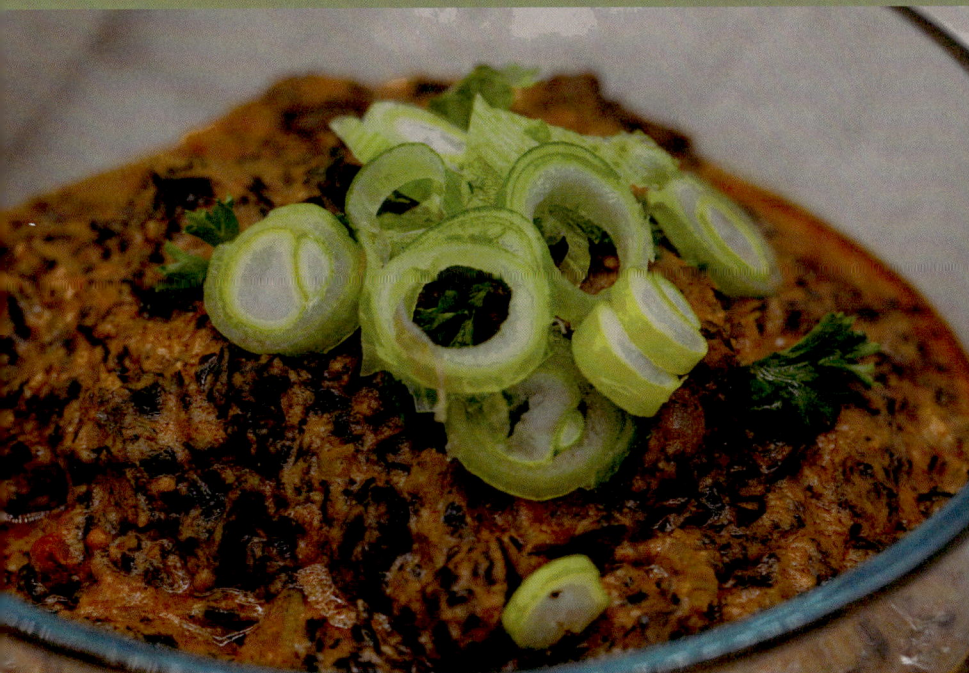

Ingredients

1 Pre cooked whole chicken
   cut in pieces (reserved
   with stock)
3 tbsp organic tomato paste
1 tbsp smoked paprika
3 tbsp organic natural peanut
   butter (creamy no sugar
   added)
1 bag frozen collard greens
   (12 0z) or more
1 tbsp of chicken bouillon
   powder
1 half medium red onion
   diced
1 tbsp diced green onion for
   garnishing
1 tsp kosher salt
3 cups water
2 tbsp garlic bell pepper base
1 tsp cayenne pepper
   (optional)

Directions

1

In a medium heated large pot, add water, peanut butter.
With a wire whisk, stir vigorously until the mixer turn
creamy. Bring the mixture to a boil for about 8 minutes or
until you see peanut butter oil make his way to the surface

2

Add Tomato paste., paprika, garlic bell pepper base base,
and cook for 5 more minute. Stir occasionally to avoid
burning at the bottom.Me while, under a cold water, rinse
the collard green in a strainer for 2 minutes and set
aside.Add the chicken in the stock, bouillon, salt, diced
onion, cayenne pepper and stir very well.

3

Boil the mixture for 5 minutes then add the collard green
and reduce to low heat and simmer for another 5 more
minutes. At this point the soup should be thick and leafy.
Taste for flavor and make adjustment if there is any.
Serve the stew over rice or any grain and garnish with green
onion. Enjoy !

*Like many other leafy green,
collard greens are excellent
sources of vitamin A, C, K
iron and calcium.*

Indian Fish Curry with Chives

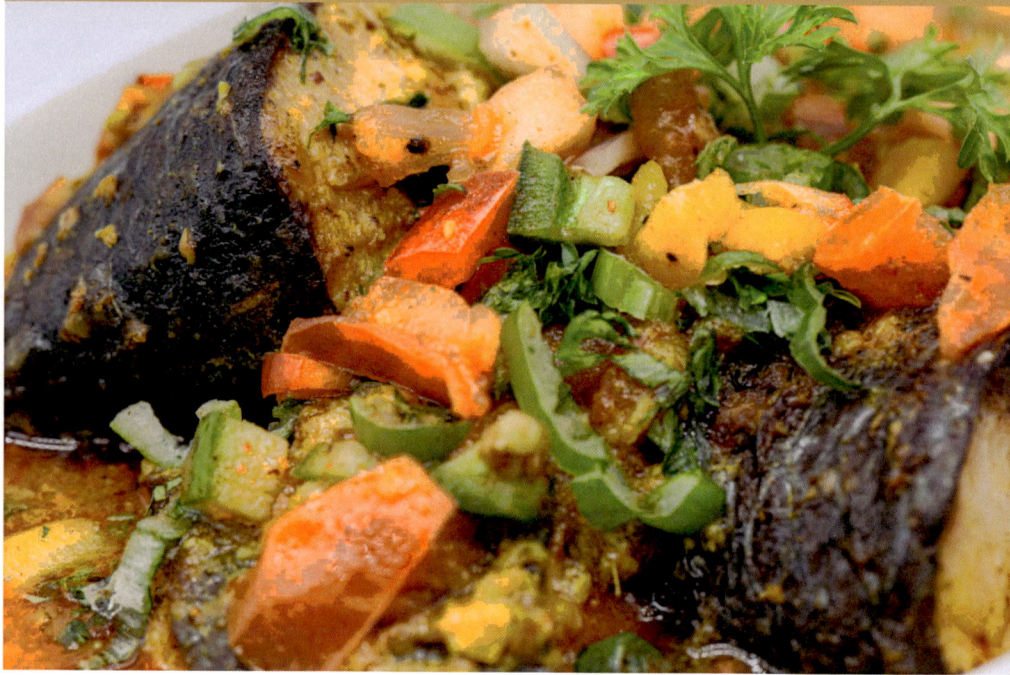

Directions

1 Mix the mustard, pepper, 1/2 teaspoon salt, and 2 tablespoons of olive oil in a shallow bowl. Add the fish fillets, turning to coat. Marinate the fish in the refrigerator for 15 minutes.

2 Combine the onion, garlic, ginger, and cashews in a blender or food processor and pulse until the mixture forms a paste.

3 Preheat an oven to 350 degrees F (175 degrees C).

4 Heat 1 tablespoon of grape seed oil in a skillet over medium-low heat. Stir in the prepared paste; cook and stir for a minute or two.

5 Add Curry powder, salt, and sugar. Cook and stir for an additional five minutes. Stir in the chopped tomato and vegetable broth.

6 Arrange the fish fillets in a baking dish, Top the fish with the sauce, cover the baking dish, and bake in the preheated oven until the fish flakes easily with a fork, about 30 minutes. Garnish with chopped cilantro.

Ingredients

For the marinade:
2 teaspoons Dijon mustard
1 teaspoon ground black pepper
1/2 teaspoon salt
seasoning bouillon or stock
2 tablespoons olive oil
4 Trunks bass fish or cod fillet
1 onion, coarsely chopped
4 cloves garlic, roughly chopped
1 (1 inch) piece fresh ginger root, peeled and chopped
5 cashew halves
1 tablespoon grape seeds oil
2 teaspoons cayenne pepper, to taste or pepper flake (optional for you if you desire most Indian foods are spicy)
Curry powder. 1 teaspoon white sugar
1/2 cup chopped tomato
1/4 cup vegetable broth
1/4 cup chopped fresh cilantro

Fish is loaded with omega-3 fatty acids and vitamins. It is also a great source of minerals such as iron iodine, potassium magnesium and zinc.

Asian Ginger Noodle Mix

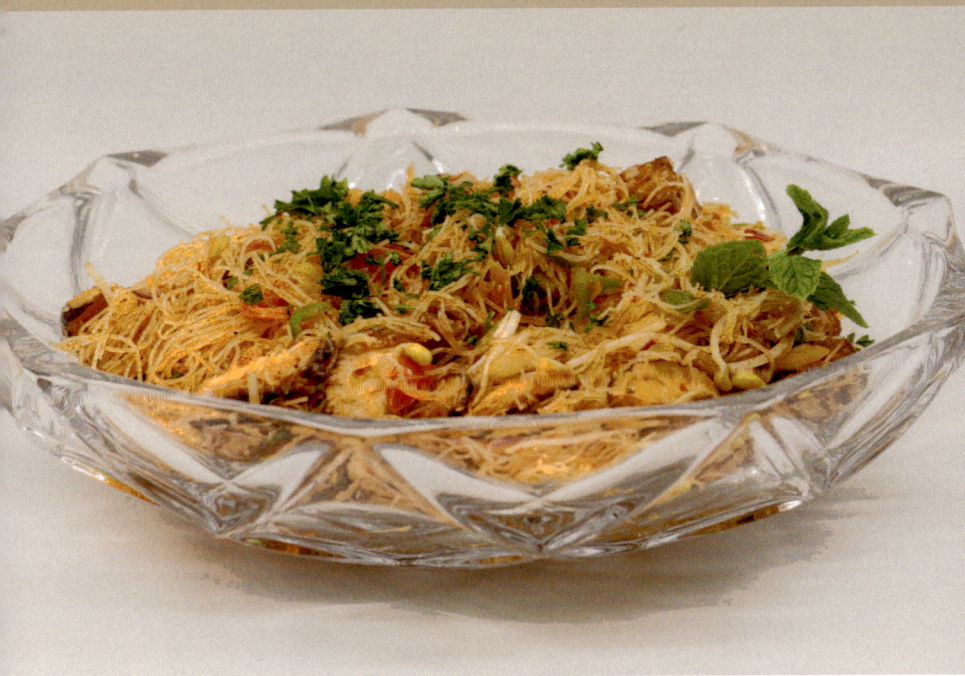

15 minutes and 4 servings

Ingredients

1 pack rice noodles (8 0Z)
1 cup crispy fried tofu cubed (optional)
2 cups bean sprouts
2 tbsp Thai chili pepper paste
2 tbsp olive oil
1 cup of cut onion
1 cup mix bell peppers (green, yellow, orange)
1 tbsp tamarin sauce
1 tsp seasoning bouillon
2 cloves garlic minced
1 tsp grated ginger
3 small slices of ginger
1 branch fresh mint
1 branch fresh curly parsley
3 cups shiitake mushroom

Directions

1.In a strainer, wash the noodle under cold water for 3 minutes or more until soften set aside.

2.Over a medium heated sauce pan, add oil, garlic, grated ginger and let it cook until the flavor is wafting.

3.Add onion, chili paste and give a good stir.

4.Add the mushroom, tamarin sauce, slices ginger, tofu and let the mix cook for 5 minutes

5.Enrich with bell peppers, bouillon powder. When the desired flavor is reached, add the noodles and stir fry for about 3 minutes until al dente.

6.Compliment with bean sprout and toss the noodle a couple of times then let it cook for another 2 minutes or until the desired softness.

7.Serve the noodle and top it with fresh parsley, garnish it with mint and enjoy!

Rice noodles are staple foods in Asian countries. They are gluten free and low in fat. Other healthy noodles to choose from include: soba noodles, quinoa noodles, sweet potato noodles and kelp noodles.

*A simple mouthwatering noodle dish.
Your family will praise you for this!*

African Jerk Chicken

1 hour 45 minutes and 3 servings

Ingredients

1 whole chicken cut into
   pieces (6 parts)
3 tbsp jerk chicken base
1 tbsp chipotle seasoning
1 tbsp chicken stock powder
1 tsp kosher salt
1 tbsp fresh shopped scallion
   (garnish)
1 bunch parsley shopped
   (garnish)
2 tbsp tamarin sauce
1 tbsp smoked paprika
¼ cup grape seed oil
2 tbsp lemon juice
1 tsp nutmeg

Directions

1 Place the chicken pieces in a large mixing bowl, add jerk base, lemon juice, salt, tamarin sauce, smoked paprika chicken stock, nutmeg and massage well until complete saturation. Marinate the chicken for 1 hour or more in the refrigerator.

2 Now preheat the oven to 375 F. Meanwhile, in a medium heat fried pan, add oil, and sauté' the chicken for 5 minutes until slightly brown on both side.

3 Now preheat the oven to 375 F. Meanwhile, in a medium heat fried pan, add oil, and sauté' the chicken for 5 minutes until slightly brown on both side.

Chicken is a lean meat and sour of protein. Therefore, it's a grea option for healthy eating. Variet of spices on this dish make it exceptional

Creamy Avocado Lumpia

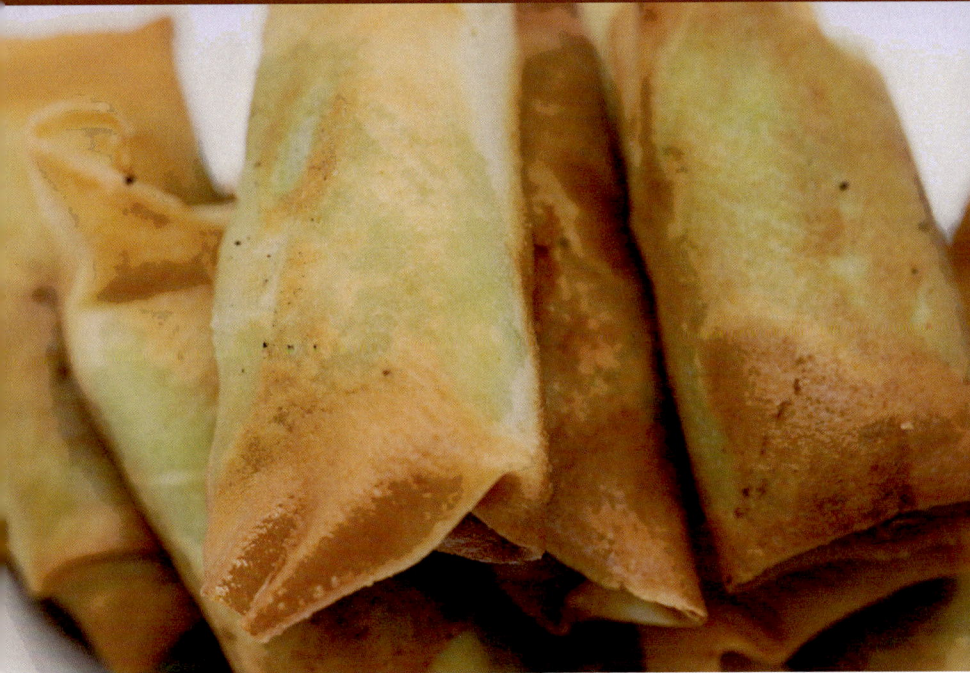

25 minutes and 6- 10 servings

Ingredients

1bag lumpia wraps
(30 wrappers)
6 ripe avocados peeled and
seeded
3 in one seasoning, dash (salt,
back pepper, and garlic
powder)
2 tbsp olive oil
¼ cup water
2 tbsp wheat flour, tapioca or
all purpose
6 cups of avocado oil or
coconut oil

*Avocado lumpias are great
appetizers. If they are made
with meat, you can freeze the
uncooked wraps and use for
another time.*

*Creamy Avocado Lumpia, just
like the name says, it will
truly melt like butter in your
mouth. Crunchy from outside,
creamy on the inside.*

Directions

1
In a small bowl, place avocados, 3 in one seasoning,
olive oil, mash with a fork until slightly creamy.
In another small bowl, mix ¼ cup water with 2 tbsp of
flour like a cold roux for sealing.
First separate the wrappers and cover with a damp
kitchen towel to prevent dryness.

2
On a clean kitchen counter, lay lumpia sheet flat but
diagonal with one point toward you.
Add 1 tbsp of avocado mix on the point facing you, roll
lumpia downward by corners and continue rolling until
you get to the very bottom of the wrapper, dip one finger
into the roux and seal the end.

3
Continue rolling until you complete the wrappers.
In a big work, over 350 F, add oil, when shimmering, add
lumpia by batches of 5 or 10 and fry them for 1-2 minutes
until brown and crispy.
Serve the avocado lumpia hot and enjoy!

African Jollof Rice & Braised Chicken

45 minutes and 6 servings

Directions

1 In a large pot, add chicken, rub the anise ginger thyme, bouillon powder, salt, 1 cup water and cook over medium-high heat for 10 minutes. Remove the chicken and set aside and reserve the stock from the chicken
In a medium frying pan, add oil and sauté the chicken until brown and crispy and set aside.

2 With the reserve stock, add bell pepper base, tomato paste and cook for 5 minutes. Add the oil from the fry pan, rosemary, curry powder, sauté' chicken, rest of water, stir well and let It boil for another 3 minutes. The sauce should be thick at this point. Scoop all the chicken out with 1 cup of the soup and set aside.

3 Now add the 4 cups of stock, onion and bring to boil. Taste the sauce and adjust the flavor if needed. Add rice, and stir thoroughly. Cover the pot with lid, reduce the heat and simmer the rice until tender and it has absorbed all the sauce for 20 minutes, but stir a few times for easy distribution of the heat and a desire for stickiness, if not skip the stirring.

4 After the 20 minutes pass, check the rice. At this point it should be soft and fluffy. Serve the rice in a bowl or plate, top it with chicken braise and then reserve sauce. Pat yourself on the back and enjoy your hard work!

Ingredients

Ingredients
3 cups Jasmine rice or brown rice
2 cups bell pepper base (sauce see pg.
3 tbsp tomato paste
4 cups chicken stock
3 cups of water
½ cups grape seed oil
1 whole chicken cut into pieces
1 tsp Kosher salt
1 tbsp bouillon powder
¼ medium onion diced
1 tbsp rosemary powder
1 tsp curry powder
2 tbsp anise ginger thyme

*Choose rice according to your health goal. Brown rice is more healthy than white rice.
In Africa, mostly jollof rice is made with white rice.
To reduce time for this dish, pre-make your sauce and chicken ahead of time, then cook the rice as pilaf rice.*

African Sautéed Golden Plantains

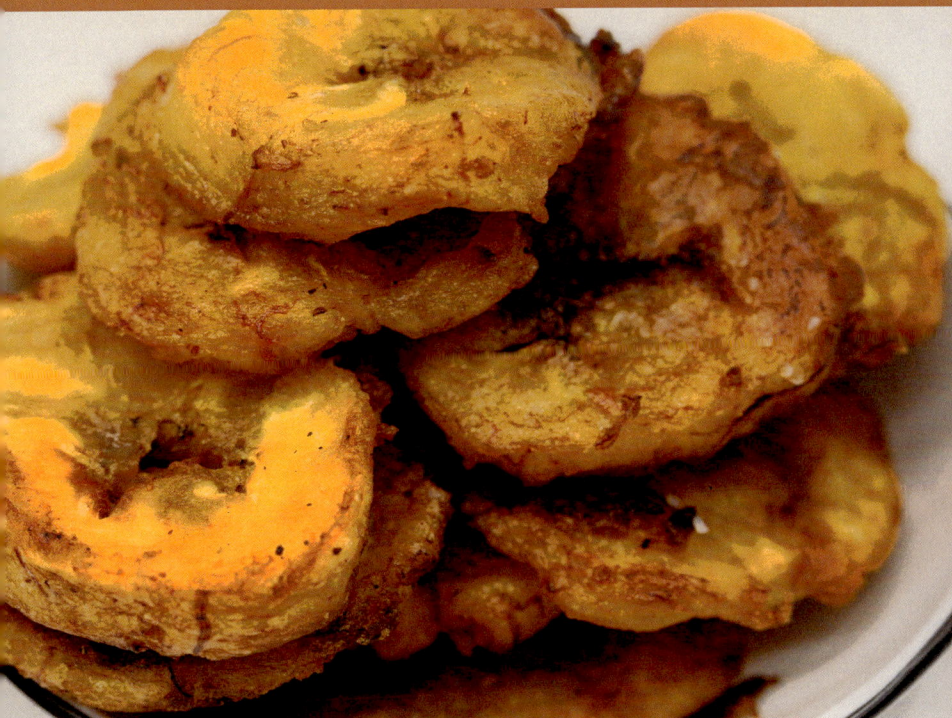

10 minutes and 3 servings

Ingredients

3 large ripened plantains
(round cut)
¼ cup grape seed oil
Dash of salt

Directions

1 In a large bowl, add plantains and dash salt, toss a few times and set aside.

2 Over medium heat, pour the oil into a nonstick skillet. When shimmering, add plantains in batches and fry for 1-2 minutes then turn to the other side and cook for another minute or until brown.

3 Remove the plantains from the skillet and drain the oil with paper towels
Continue the process until you finish frying all the plantains. Serve and enjoy

In my home country, Togo, we eat plantains sometimes with a special hot sauce called "yebese" (see page)
If you like hot and spicy go head and give it a try!

Plantains are staple foods in most tropical countries. They are a power house to complex carbohydrates, minerals and vitamins. They also can be boiled like potatoes.

African Flavorsome Shakshuka

Ingredients

5-8 large eggs
2 tbsp tomato paste
2 cups diced tomato or
    crushed (fire roasted)
1 tsp salt
1 tsp black pepper
1 tsp bouillon seasoning
1 Medium red onion diced
2 tbsp shopped parsley
    (garnish)
½ cayenne pepper (optional)
1 tsp smoked Paprika
2 cloves garlic grated
1 red pepper diced
2 tbsp olive oil

Eggs are the key ingredient for this dish, rich in selenium, minerals, and vitamins. Eggs are a complete protein.

Shakshuka "aka" Mixture in Arabic, is a dish made with tomato and eggs poached. It is rich in spices and flavor. From North Africa all the way to Israel.

Directions

1 In a medium heat over a large skillet, add oil and let it shimmering for 30 second, then add garlic, onion , sauté for 2-3 minutes until translucent .
Add tomato paste, bell pepper, smoked paprika, cayenne pepper cook for 3 minutes but stir constantly.

2 Pour the crushed or diced tomato over the mixture, add salt, bouillon seasoning and stir well. Reduce the heat and let the sauce simmer about 4 minutes. With a narrow spatula, make a hole or well around the perimeter of the skillet crack the eggs one at a time into the sauce.

3 Sprinkle black pepper and a dash of salt all over the eggs. Cover the skillet with a lid and cook for 6-8 minutes. At this point, the eggs white should be opaque and the yoks a little bit hard but jiggling in the middle. Turn the stove off, sprinkle fresh parsley and serve shakshuka with pita bread or any bread of your choice. It can also be eating alone or over rice. Enjoy!

Healthy Granola Bars

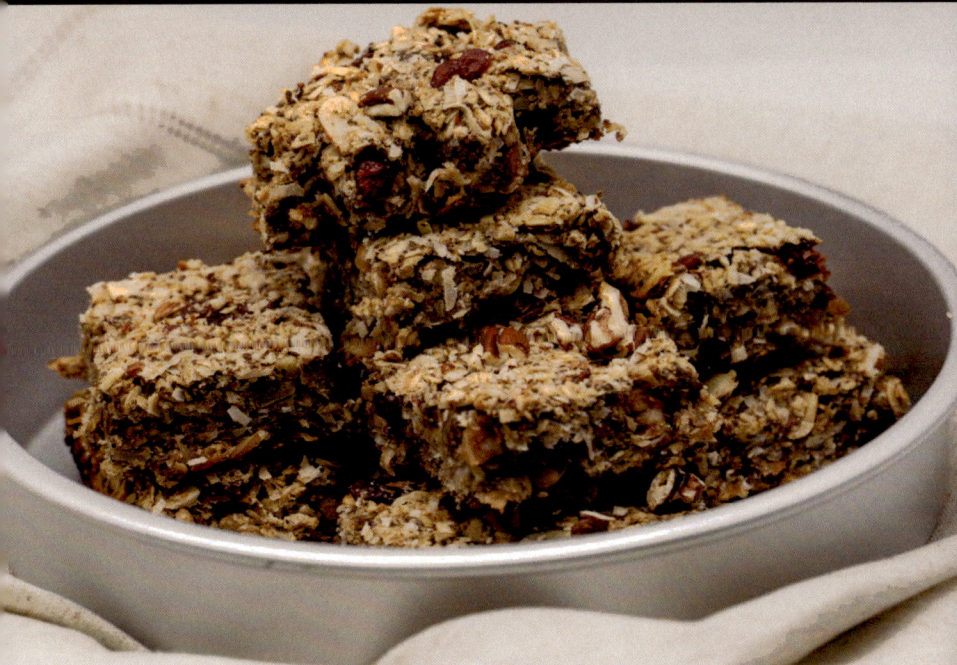

50 minutes -1 hour and 10
servings

Ingredients

4 cups whole grain rolled oats
1 cup instant quick oat
2 cups dried cranberries
1 cup pumpkin seeds
1 cup shredded coconut
1 cup chia seed
½ cup flax seed meal
3 medium bananas or 2 large
2 cups dates
2 cups shredded pineapple
½ cup of grapeseed oil or
    coconut oil
½ cup almond
½ cup pecan
1 tsp baking powder
½ kosher salt
Savory paste (sweet paste for
    the granola)
3 tbsp chunky organic peanut
    butter
1 tbsp vanilla extract
1 tsp nutmeg

Directions

1 To make the savory paste, in a blender, add dates, banana, pineapple, vanilla and blend at a creamy consistency. In a sauce pan over medium heat, add oil, peanut butter, and simmer for 2 minutes until the peanut butter gets liquified. Remove from the heat and set aside.

2 In a large mixing bowl, add oats, chia seed, dried cranberries, pumpkin seeds, shredded coconut, flax seed, almond, pecans, salt, baking powder, and give a good stir. Pour the savory and the peanut butter and mix well until all combined. The mixture should be wet and slightly sticky.

3 Turn the oven to 325 F, in a 9x9 inch baking pan with parchment paper, press the granola firmly and evenly into the baking pan. With a flat dough scraper, smooth all the corners of the pan and top. Bake the granola for 30 minutes but check it a couple of times to make sure they are not burning on top. After it's done, remove from oven and let it cool off for 5 minutes, then cut into bar shapes. Serve the granola and enjoy!

Oats are one of the healthiest grains on the planet. Rich in fiber, minerals, vitamins and antioxidants.

75

STAY CONNECTED

@chef_Malaika

@Les-Graines-de-Vie-Holistic-Health-Wellness

Don't miss a single thing! Sign up for my monthly news letter to receive monthly watering recipes and health tips.

www.lesgrainesdevie.com/newsletter

This book was inspired by my experience at the Institute for Integrative Nutrition® (IIN), where I received my training in holistic wellness and health coaching.
IIN offers a truly comprehensive Health Coach Training Program that invites students to deeply explore the things that are most nourishing to them. From the physical aspects of nutrition and eating wholesome foods that work best for each individual person, to the concept of Primary Food – the idea that everything in life, including our spirituality, career, relationships, and fitness contributes to our inner and outer health – IIN helped me reach optimal health and balance. This inner journey unleashed the passion that compels me to share what I've learned and inspire others.
Beyond personal health, IIN offers training in health coaching, as well as business and marketing. Students who choose to pursue this field professionally complete the program equipped with the communication skills and branding knowledge they need to create a fulfilling career encouraging and supporting others in reaching their own health goals.
From renowned wellness experts as Visiting Teachers to the convenience of their online learning platform, this school has changed my life, and I believe it will do the same for you. I invite you to learn more about the Institute for Integrative Nutrition and explore how the Health Coach Training Program can help you transform your life. Feel free to contact me to hear more about my personal experience at www.LesGrainesdeVie.com/integrativenutrition or call (844) 315-8546 to learn more.

Did you enjoy my book? I would love a review! Please give me you honest feedback on Amazon.

"Too Busy To Cook"

Unleashing Your Inner Culinary Skills.

"Let thy food be thy medicine, and medicine be thy food"
-Hippocrates

- Do you feel overwhelmed with cooking?
- Do you always feel like you never have time to cook?
- Do you often go out to eat?

Les Graines de Vie
HOLISTIC HEALTH & WELLNESS

Malaika Bagoudou is a Health Coach, Personal Chef; and author. She received training from the Institute for Integrative Nutrition. Malaika works with busy Men and women and their families who are ready to take their health to the next level. Clients describe her as "inspiring" and motivating." For more information on Malaika or to stay in the know, visit www.LesGrainesdeVie.com

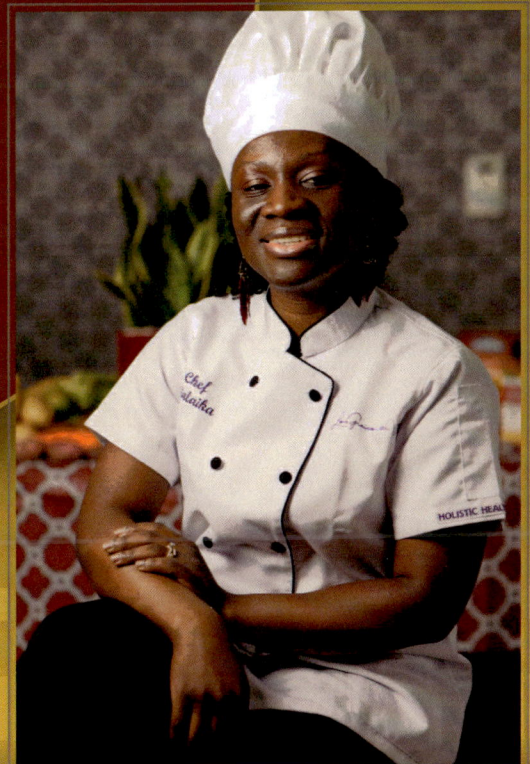

BENEFITS OF THIS BOOK:

. Make quick healthy foods that will nourish your body

. Unleashing your culinary skills

. Prioritize your health and wellness

. Eating on a low budget

. Save time in the kitchen

ISBN 978-1-7347687-0-1
$29.99
52999>

9 781734 768701